HEALTH

AS EXPANDING

CONSCIOUSNESS

MARGARET A. NEWMAN

Ph.D., R.N., F.A.A.N.

Professor, School of Nursing
University of Minnesota
Minneapolis, Minnesota

Supplement by

JOANNE M. MARCHIONE, M.A., R.N.

Associate Professor, College of Nursing
University of Akron, Akron, Ohio

The C. V. Mosby Company

ST. LOUIS • WASHINGTON, D.C. • TORONTO • 1986

MOSBY

A TRADITION OF PUBLISHING EXCELLENCE

Editor: Tom Lochhaas
Assistant editor: Maureen Slaten
Project editor: Sylvia Kluth
Manuscript editor: Peggy Fagen
Book design: Gail Morey Hudson
Production: Florence Fansher

Printed in the United States of America

The C.V. Mosby Company
11830 Westline Industrial Drive, St. Louis, Missouri 63146

Library of Congress Cataloging-in-Publication Data

Newman, Margaret A.
  Health as expanding consciousness.

  Bibliography: p.
  1. Family—Health and hygiene.   2. Nursing.
I. Title. [DNLM: 1. Consciousness—nurses' instruction.
2. Family—nurses' instruction.   3. Health Promotion—methods
—nurses' instruction.   WA 590 N554h]
RA418.5.F3N48   1986   613   86-16334
ISBN 0-8016-3693-0

UE/VH/VH   9 8 7 6 5 4 3 2 1   02/D/278

TO

MY MOTHER

Mamie Love Donald Newman

who taught me
to dance and make music
and in the experience of her illness
to let go
live in the present
and love

AND

MY FATHER

Ivo Mathias Newman

who helped me experience
the fun of numbers
the neatness of logic
and the company of contemplation

Life has to be in the moment,
spontaneous and vulnerable.
There isn't any winning or losing.
Life itself . . . is the reward
and isn't always easy or fun . . .
the issue of happiness is irrelevant.
The relevant quest is the
expansion of consciousness.

Richard Moss
The I That is We

CONTENTS

CONTENTS

HEALTH
AS EXPANDING
CONSCIOUSNESS

INTRODUCTION

Intuition plays a large part in my life. The books I have chosen to read, the people I have met, the jobs I have taken, the places where I have lived, all somehow fit together in a pattern that is right for me. Sometimes I have been able to sense the pattern well in advance of its coming together. Other times I just plunge ahead because it feels right. Even seeming mistakes turn out all right in the long run, once you realize there is no such thing as a mistake. Every experience of life is a gift, to be claimed and learned from.

I learned early in life that things do not always—or hardly ever—turn out the way you want and that you have a choice: You can be miserable because of it, or you can find a way to make a miserable experience meaningful and even enjoyable. I decided to pursue the latter.

The most pronounced of my early experiences was my mother's nine-year struggle with amyotrophic lateral sclerosis, a degenerative disease of the motor neurons. Her early symptoms began as I was finishing high school and progressed to partial incapacitation during the years I was away at college, almost unnoticed by me as I was struggling to establish my identity as a young adult. However, once I was back home after graduation from college, I was confronted with the unmistakable dependence of my mother on my brother, my sister-in-law, and me. I won't go into the details of the professional help we did and did not have, or the agony of the decisions we had to make, or the frustration caused by the infringement of my mother's illness on our lives. I *do* want to share my realization that life had to be lived in the present and that if one was to be happy, it had to come one day at a time. I learned that my mother, though physically incapacitated, was not really "ill." She was a person, a whole person, just like anyone else. I came to know her and to love her in a way that probably never would have occurred had she not been physically dependent. The five years I spent with her before she died were difficult, tiring, and restrictive in some ways but intense, loving, and expanding in other ways. As another person has described it, I have faced great difficulty and have come through it. I had the feeling then that I was preparing for something else.

I had been feeling a call to nursing as a career for a number of years. When I went to Baylor, a Southern Baptist university, in 1950, I had no idea what direction my life would take. I was caught up in the religious fervor of my surroundings for several years, and true to the predominant values of the early fifties, I thought the ideal goal for my life was to be a conscientious and devoted wife. A gnawing conscience-like feeling began to haunt me during my junior year and never left me alone for very long after that: the feeling that I should become a nurse. There couldn't have been a worse prospect as far as I was concerned! Nursing represented all the things I did not like: illness, hospitals, needles, and so on. The things I did like, however— math, music, art, dance—did not seem to lead the way to a career for me.

When my mother died, I had just uttered a prayer of willingness to follow that lingering call to nursing. Within two weeks I was enrolled at the University of Tennessee School of Nursing in Memphis.

I knew, after only a few classes, that nursing was right for me. Contrary to my earlier projections, nursing focused on the complexity of human beings in health and illness, something I had experienced with my mother. I realized that nursing was going to demand the best of my intellect as well as the utmost of my humanity. After graduation I went almost directly into graduate study, and under the tutelage of a very sensitive, intelligent teacher, I began to articulate a synthesis of my experience and learning in terms of the essence of the illness experience and what nursing had to offer. Basic among these learnings was that illness reflected the life pattern of the person and that what was needed was the recognition of that pattern and acceptance of it for what it meant to that person.

Years later, I came to the conclusion that **health is the expansion of consciousness**. It frightens me to think I might have missed that revelation, for it is so important to me now. But even my fear is unwarranted, because one can trust the evolving pattern—it is a pattern of evolving, expanding consciousness *regardless* of the form or direction it takes. Because of this realization illness and disease have lost their demoralizing power. I want to share this realization. We are in the wonderful process of expanding consciousness, of things becoming clearer, of moving from "seeing through a glass darkly" to knowing as we are known.

And there is so much more. The expansion of consciousness never ends. In this way aging has lost its power. Death has lost its power. There is peace and meaning in suffering. We are free from all the things we have feared—loss, death, dependency. We can let go of fear.

Throughout my career as an acknowledged theorist, I have been involved, if not embroiled, in the controversy of what is science and what is scientific. In order to side-step that issue here, I would like to say at the outset that this book is not necessarily about science but rather about *meaning*: the meaning of life and of health and of what those of us in the health professions can do about it. Ken Wilbur (1983) has captured the point in these statements:

> While we will not shun empirical data (that would miss the point), neither will we confine ourselves to empirical data (that would miss the point completely). (p. 33)
>
> A physician can describe the intricate biochemical processes that constitute your living being: he [sic] can to some extent repair them, cure them of disease, and operate to remove malfunctions. But he cannot then tell you the *meaning* of that life whose every working mechanism he understands. (p. 2)

The meaning of life and health, I submit, will be found in the evolving process of expanding consciousness.

This book is about a different way of viewing health and disease—a new paradigm. It is grounded in my own personal experience but was stimulated by Martha Rogers' insistence on the unitary nature of a human being in interaction with the environment (Rogers, 1970). While a student in Martha's seminar, I was intrigued, and plagued, by her statement that health and illness are "simply" expressions of the life process—one no more important than the other. How could that be? Possibly they are opposite ends of a continuum. No, she said. How about opposite sides of a coin? No, she said.

I continued to struggle with this idea. A few years later, in a conference with a graduate student about rhythmic phenomena, I had an "Aha" that revealed health and illness as a single process and, like rhythmic phenomena, becoming manifest in ups and downs, or peaks and troughs, moving through varying degrees of organization and disorganization, but all as one unitary process. Later my previous introduction to the antagonistic but complementary forces of order and disorder, so essential to our continuing development as self-organizing creatures, became more understandable within the context of health and disease.

Then I became acquainted with Itzhak Bentov's work, which provided logical explanations for many things I had taken on faith up to that point (Bentov, 1978). For instance, Teilhard de Chardin's belief that a person's consciousness continues to develop beyond the physical life and becomes a part of a universal consciousness had made sense to me (Teilhard de Chardin, 1959). Not only was it consistent with my Christian belief of life after death, but it just seemed reasonable that one would not spend a lifetime developing the knowledge and wisdom of one's total being (consciousness) and then have it dissipate into nothing. It made more sense that it continue to develop and join with a larger consciousness.

Bentov's explanations of the evolution of consciousness were matter-of-fact and almost "scientific." They were logical and down to earth. I had the opportunity to hear Bentov speak and to participate in a workshop led by him about that time, and I was convinced that this spontaneous, unassuming man *knew* what he was talking about. When accused of talking about religion, he replied, "No, I'm talking about knowledge." When asked how he knew these things, he said, "I just know." What he said felt right. There comes a time when one seeks knowledge that is more than the observable facts.

David Bohm's theory of implicate order helped me to put these thoughts and experiences into perspective (Bohm, 1980). I began to comprehend the underlying, unseen pattern that manifests itself in varying forms, including disease, and the interconnectedness and omnipresence of all that there is.

Arthur Young's theory of human evolution pinpoints the crucial role of insight, or pattern recognition, in the process

(Young, 1976a, 1976b) and was the impetus for my efforts to integrate the basic concepts of my theory—movement, space, time, and consciousness—into a dynamic portrayal of life and health. Richard Moss's experience of love as the highest level of consciousness provided affirmation and elaboration of my intuition regarding the nature of health (Moss, 1981).

As I sit here in awe and feel inadequate to the task of synthesizing these ideas in a meaningful way, I wonder how I could feel otherwise.

CHAPTER 1

A NEW PARADIGM OF HEALTH

The view that health is the absence of disease has pervaded most of our thinking from very early in life. From the immunizations that prevent devastating childhood diseases to admonitions to brush our teeth and drink our milk, the predominant view is that health (absence of disease) is within our control, and it is our responsibility to make sure we have it. This view is so strong that those who don't have it are viewed as inferior or even repulsive and don't belong with the responsible majority who have exercised the appropriate self-control with its concomitant (or so they think) perfect health. Indeed those who are labeled with a serious disease often question what they have done to deserve this fate or worry about whether or not their family will be able to continue to accept them in their diseased state.

The way we talk about health, one would think it is a commodity that can be purchased. We say we can promote it and deliver it. We advise everyone to make sure they have it or get it, because apparently it is possible to lose it. We criticize those who do things that we consider destroy it, and we even go so far as to disassociate ourselves from them.

We have become idolatrous of health. We have created places of worship of health at which we carry out the recommended rituals to obtain or maintain health. Then when one of the leading gurus dies while engaging in one of these rituals, we say in its defense, "How much sooner would he have died if he had not engaged in it"—as if death were the antithesis of health, or the ultimate put-down.

There have been many attempts to get away from the notion of health as the absence of disease. Dunn (1959) was perhaps the first to use the term "high-level wellness" and to portray health on a continuum from wellness to illness. Later he defined health as "an integrated method of functioning . . . oriented toward maximizing the potential of which the individual is capable" (Dunn, 1973, p. 7). Dubos (1965), another health spokesperson of the sixties, characterized health as the adaptive potential of an individual. He was referring primarily to adaptation to environmental challenges. Others have viewed health in terms of normality, life-style, and conformity to social norms (Ardell, 1977; Dolfman, 1973; Parsons, 1958).

Although the authors of these concepts tend to reject the idea of health as the absence of disease, a prevailing notion throughout the health literature is the seeking and accomplishment of a disease-free state. A well-known contemporary, Lewis Thomas (1979), is probably the most explicit in this respect and is convinced that a disease-free state will eventually be accomplished through the work of medical scientists. At the time of this writing, a featured article on genetic engineering appearing in a Sunday newspaper magazine section set forth the claim, "Scientists explore the promise of tomorrow—a world without disease" (Ubell, 1985). The prevailing views of health, then, might be categorized as ranging from:

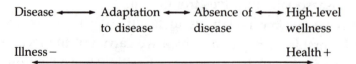

This portrayal dichotomizes health and illness. Health is the positive state to be desired. Illness (disease) is the negative state. Even though many of the high-level wellness theorists speak of health and illness as integrated, dynamic concepts, a polarization is maintained as one strives for the positive state identified with health and avoids the negative state identified with disease.

There is another view. For a number of years I have been saying that disease is a manifestation of health. This view requires another approach. Certainly we no longer would say we want to promote health (as disease). Those of us in the health care field have devoted most of our careers to preventing disease, or getting rid of it when it occurs, or, for some of us, ignoring it and hoping it will go away.

So how can I say that disease is health? To do this one has to reject a dichotomous or polarized view of health and disease and think in terms of a synthesized view based on a dialectical fusion of opposites: One point of view fuses with the opposite point of view and brings forth a new, synthesized view.

In this case, "disease" fuses with its opposite, absence of disease, "nondisease," and brings forth a new concept of "health":

Disease–Nondisease⟶Health

This synthesized view incorporates disease as a meaningful aspect of health. Jantsch (1980) goes further and asserts that process thinking transcends a synthesis of opposites, leaving only complementarity, in which the opposites include each other. This would mean that health includes disease *and* disease includes health. Both of these ways of thinking are echoed by Bohm (1981):

> When you trace a particular absolute notion to what appears to be its logical conclusion, you find it to be identical with its opposite, and therefore the whole dualism collapses, as Hegel found. Reason first shows you that opposites pass into each other, then you discover that one opposite reflects the other, and finally you find that they are identical to each other—not really different at all. (p. 31)

Whichever way one chooses to look at it, the important consideration is that disease is a meaningful aspect of the whole.

ELIMINATING DICHOTOMIES

Rogers' conceptualization of a unitary being eliminated the usual dichotomy between health and disease (Rogers, 1970). She pointed out that health and illness should be viewed equally as expressions of the life process and that the meaning of these phenomena is derived from an understanding of the life process in its totality. Rogers' early critics considered such a view unscientific; however, an increasingly large number of scientists and philosophers are recognizing the limitations of a quantitative, analytical approach, especially as it relates to the life process and health of human beings, and are calling for a qualitative, intuitive recognition of the total patterning of a person.

One of the difficulties in relinquishing a dichotomous view of health and disease is our fragmentary way of thinking and talking. It is easy for us to think of disease separately from health and to proceed to attend to it as a separate part. Dividing things into parts is useful, but eventually it becomes more than just a way of thinking about things: it becomes reality itself. We begin to think of disease as separate from the person it occupies and from the world within and around the person. Our language reinforces this separatism and promotes the idea that one object can act on another object, such as a virus acting on a person or objects interacting with each other—still with the idea of each being a separate, independent entity. This view is no longer sufficient to explain the reality of our world.

Science is demanding a nonfragmentary world view. Experiments at the particle level demonstrate that two particles separated in space display correlated movements simultaneously, indicating "that the various particles have to be taken literally as projections of a higher-dimensional reality which cannot be accounted for in terms of any force of interaction between them" (Bohm, 1980, pp. 186–187). To illustrate, David Bohm suggests envisioning projections of two television cameras focused on the same phenomenon from different angles.

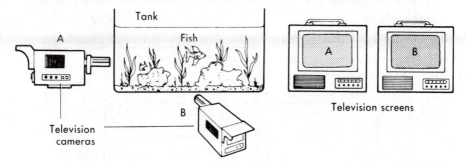

Fig. 1 Reprinted with permission from Bohm, D. (1980). *Wholeness and the implicate order*. London: Routledge & Kegan Paul, p. 187.

Projection A and projection B contain images that move at the same time and are somehow related, but there is no interaction between the two and neither portrays the whole picture. Rather, they are manifestations in two-dimensional form of a phenomenon of greater dimensions.

The two projections are different points of view of the same larger reality. Now substitute mind and body for projections A and B.

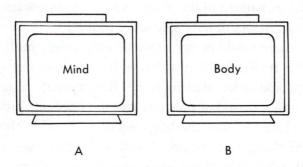

Fig. 2

In the same way, mind and body are manifestations of the same larger reality. Contrary to previous thinking, one does not cause the other or control the other, as in "mind over matter" terminology, but each is a reflection of an underlying pattern of a phenomenon of greater dimensions. Each is reflective of the larger whole.

Now take this point of view one step further. Substitute disease and nondisease for projections A and B.

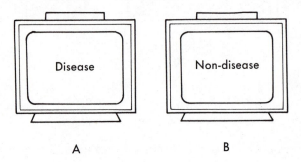

Fig. 3

Disease and nondisease are each reflections of the larger whole. Reconsideration of the original synthesis of health and disease yields a new concept: *pattern of the whole.*

A PARADIGM OF PATTERN

Health as pattern of the whole is a point of view consistent with Bohm's theory of implicate order (Bohm, 1980). According to Bohm, there exists in our universe an unseen, multidimensional pattern that is the ground, or basis, for all things. This is the implicate order. Arising out of the implicate order is the explicate order, a kind of precipitate of the implicate order. The explicate order includes the tangibles of our world. These tangibles—the things we can see, touch, hear, feel—are so much more real to us than the underlying unseen pattern that we think the explicate order is primary, the real thing. Actually, according to Bohm, the implicate order is primary. The explicate order arises periodically from the implicate, like waves appearing and disappearing on the surface of the ocean. The explicate, whatever form it may take, is a temporary manifestation of a total undivided pattern.

In the context of the theory of implicate order, *health, encompassing disease and nondisease, can be regarded as the explication of the underlying pattern of the person-environment.* Observable phenomena—such as body temperature, blood pressure, and heart rate; neoplasms and biochemical variations; diet and exercise; communication—are all manifestations of person-environment interaction. Viewing these manifestations as reflections of the underlying pattern makes it possible for us to *see* the pattern and thereby begin to understand it.

The essence of the emerging paradigm of health is pattern recognition. It involves moving from looking at parts to looking at patterns. The pattern is information that depicts the whole, understanding of the meaning of all the relationships at once. It is a fundamental attribute of all there is and gives unity in diversity (Rogers, 1970).

An understanding of pattern has become increasingly basic to an understanding of health. Health has been defined in terms of patterns of energy exchange (Roy et al., 1982). From the moment we are conceived to the moment we die, in spite of changes that accompany aging, we manifest a pattern that identifies us as a particular person: the genetic pattern that contains information that directs our becoming, the voice pattern that is recognizable across distances and over time, the movement pattern that identifies a person known to us a long way off even though no other features can be seen. These patterns are among the many explicate manifestations of the underlying pattern. It is the pattern of our lives that identifies us, not the substances that go into making up that pattern. Ability to comprehend the concept of unitary human beings is enhanced as the concept of pattern is understood.

What is pattern? How can we get a hold on it? For one thing, it is relatedness. Characteristics of patterning include movement, diversity and rhythm. The pattern is in constant movement or change, the parts are diverse and are changing in relation to each other, and rhythm identifies the pattern. Pattern or patterning is somehow intimately involved in energy exchange and transformation. As energy is exchanged, relationships within the pattern change. We become aware of pattern via waves of energy: the pictures we perceive through variations in light waves and the music we sense in terms of sound waves.

The ground or background of particular forms is equally as important as the form itself. We are able to recognize patterns by variations in contrast, e.g., the many subtleties of light and dark or of loud and soft. If the contrast is too slight or occurs over an extended period, we may not be sensitive to the pattern.

Sometimes the pattern cannot be seen all at once. For example, Bohm, in describing the underlying pattern of the implicate order, suggests imagining a drop of ink placed in glycerin between two concentric cylinders. If the cylinders are rotated so that the particles of ink are distributed throughout the glycerin, becoming invisible, the pattern might be considered implicit (enfolded). The particles are there, nevertheless, and will reappear (become explicit or unfolded) when the cylinders are rotated in the opposite direction. Bohm elaborates: "The particle is only an abstraction that is manifest to our senses. *What is* is always a totality of ensembles, all present to-

gether, in an orderly series of stages of enfoldment and un-
foldment, which intermingle and interpenetrate each other in
principle throughout the whole of space" (Bohm, 1980, p. 184).
We need to remind ourselves that our manifest reality is a small
portion of the total enfoldment of the pattern in time-space.

Extending the time frame helps to reveal the pattern. The
field of chronobiology demonstrates the importance of viewing
phenomena over time. A body temperature that might appear
to be "abnormal" if recorded at only one time of the day may
represent merely the peak of a normal cycle or the turning point
in the healing processes underway. So it is with other phenomena that may appear to be disruptive at the time of their occur-
rence but, if viewed within an extended time frame, represent
the reorganizing activity that precedes a higher level of organization.

Seeing the pattern is facilitated by stepping out of the system, as when one views a maze from above. This perspective
eliminates the duality of separate objects, which, from a high-
level view, are dispensable. That pattern, in turn, may constitute a part of another pattern at an even higher level of
organization. This latter point can be seen when one switches
from viewing the pattern of a person to the pattern of the family
of which the person is a part, or further to the pattern of a
community, and so on.

The whole of a person or of a universe is a pattern in which
the parts cannot stand alone as separate. Entities, in and of
themselves, provide only limited understanding. They are fic-
tions of language, or of our mental models, for the purpose of
figuring and describing. The important factor is the *relationship*
between the entities: the self-regulating transformation by
which the parts are continually being articulated into an ever

changing whole. The changing pattern of a kaleidoscope is a good way to visualize this phenomenon.

Viewed from the perspective of the larger pattern, the activity of individual parts is understood in terms of the activity of the total system. Clusters of alliances among the parts change in relation to the tasks that need to be done. When one comprehends the whole, knowledge of the parts becomes meaningful. When one understands the configuration which is a triangle, knowledge of two sides and an angle gives one knowledge of the whole.

The paradox, then, is that the whole can be seen in the parts. A specific event can be viewed as an example of a class of events, and in this way the most specific patterns of a person may serve as prototypes of the general overall pattern of the person. There is generality in the specific. When an expert clinician monitors a pulse, she or he perceives much more about the person than merely the number of heartbeats per minute. In the same way a person's manner of walking communicates much more about his or her general well-being and relationship to the world than simply the number of steps taken per minute or the amount of space traversed. This assumption, that the whole can be seen in the part, is basic to the process of diagnosis of the whole (Newman, 1984). The important thing to keep in mind is the search for the unitary pattern.

The inability to discern pattern, such as when the pattern is irregular or erratic, is important and may reveal a process of reorganization or a cue to search for the larger pattern of which it is a part. An observation may represent two or more meanings at different levels of organization. Considering that the explicate manifestation of reality is a limited view of the larger multidimensional reality, we need to be attuned to the fact that the pattern we glimpse is in the process of unfolding.

THE PARADIGM SHIFT

Ferguson (1980) outlines the paradigm shift taking place in regard to health. Several of the changes are particularly relevant to the point being made here: that disease is a meaningful aspect of health. The shift is from treatment of symptoms to a search for *patterns*; from viewing pain and disease as wholly negative to a view that pain and disease are *information*; from seeing the body as a machine in good or bad repair to seeing the body as a *dynamic field of energy* within other fields; from seeing disease as an entity to seeing it as a *process*.

This paradigm shift is apparent in the nursing literature. The majority of the conceptual models have been based on a view of the patient as a person in good or bad repair and needing more or less help from nursing to regain or attain a state referred to as maximum health or well-being. Rogers' (1970) view represented a turning point in the conceptualization of person-environment interaction. The absence of boundaries between person and environment and the emphasis on mutual simultaneous interaction of person-environment demands a nondichotomous view. Rogers' insistence on a unitary view of the pattern of person-environment forces one to view the emerging pattern as a whole and as part of a greater whole.

The old paradigm is an instrumental paradigm. One identifies what is wrong in a system and tries to fix it.

The new paradigm is relational. The pattern of relationships is paramount. The task is not to try to change another person's pattern but to recognize it and relate to it in an authentic way.

The instrumental paradigm is linear, causal, predictive, dichotomous, rational, empirical, quantitative, and controlling. The relational paradigm is patterned, acausal, probabilistic, unitary, intuitive, qualitative, and innovative. But before I fall into the trap of dichotomizing, I must remind myself and the reader that a new paradigm incorporates the old paradigm and extends it. When Copernicus introduced the view of the universe with the sun, rather than the earth, as the center, his view retained the phenomena of the old view but explained them from a different standpoint. The shift in paradigms from Newtonian physics to Einsteinian and further to quantum theory presents a broader, more complete explanation of phenomena but re-affirms the old relationships under certain conditions. Therefore it is important to think of the characteristics of the old paradigm of health as special cases of the new. Viewed within the context of pattern, information from the old paradigm will have new meaning.

Within the new paradigm, pattern recognition is the essence of practice. Pattern recognition is the heart of human interaction. It is basic to responding to the individuality of another person and therefore basic to the health professional's effective use of self in therapeutic interaction. What we sense in terms of pattern is a function of our own level of awareness, sensitivity to self, and point of view.

The patterns of interaction of person-environment constitute health. The emphasis on health as process implies movement toward something. The meaning of this process differs slightly from author to author: increasing complexity, growth, transformation, evolution of consciousness. Embedded within all of these concepts is the idea that events that may appear to be undesirable, such as disease or disability, are part of a much larger, meaningful process. By interacting with the event, no matter how destructive the force might seem to be, its energy augments our own and enhances our power in the situation. In order to see this, it is necessary to grasp the pattern of the whole.

CHAPTER 2

DISEASE AS PATTERN:

DISEASE AS HEALTH

Viewing disease as health is a revolutionary idea. The term "revolutionary" means a sudden, radical, or complete change; a rotation, or about-face; a turning point. A radical change in our point of view is needed in order to eliminate the dichotomizing of health and disease that is so prevalent. Disease has been regarded as the enemy, that may strike anywhere at any time. The person who is stricken is the victim and has little to say about the situation. The troops that fight disease are led by the medical armament. These commonly used metaphors are illustrative of the way in which our language reinforces disease as the enemy to be overcome and as an entity separate from ourselves.

An increasing number of people concerned with health are recognizing the failure of this frontal attack on disease in bringing about significant changes in our sense of health and well-being (Capra, 1982; Pelletier, 1985). Relating the efforts of modern medicine to Bohm's theory of implicate order, Dossey (1982) states:

> They focus only on the reality of the explicate order, the realm of our habitation, where the world is one of separate objects and events. The implicate domain, where the very *meaning* of health, disease, and death radically changes, is currently of no concern to medicine. (p. 189)

An about-face is needed in our attitude toward disease. We need to see disease not as a separate entity that invades our bodies but as a manifestation of the pattern of person-environment interaction that identifies each of us as a unique pattern of consciousness within a field of absolute consciousness.

RHYTHMIC FLUCTUATIONS

A number of years ago, when I was contemplating one of the theories related to biological rhythms, I began to conceptualize health and illness in terms of the fluctuating pattern of rhythmic phenomena. It seemed to me that there are times when the pattern of a person becomes increasingly disharmonious, similar to when one's physiological rhythms are out of phase. This situation can continue until the person becomes what is ordinarily regarded as sick. The sickness then can provide a kind of shock that reorganizes the relationships of the person's pattern in a more harmonious way. Consider the function of a high fever, or an emotional crisis, or the accident that occurs at a particularly crucial time. These and many other critical incidents often provide the shock that facilitates the person's jump from one pattern to another, presumably at a higher level of development. So, if we view illness as something discrete, something to be avoided, diminished, or eliminated altogether, we may be ruling out the very factor that can bring about the change in the life process that the person is naturally seeking. Illness may accomplish for people what they secretly want but are not able to acknowledge, even to themselves. Ferguson (1980) has pointed out that people who get sick don't want to be their "old self" again; she described a woman who had had a stroke and who "conceded that she hadn't faced the fact that she wanted to change her life. So the stroke changed her life" (p. 252).

If we understood the patterns of our lives, then perhaps we would be in a position to maintain harmonious relationships without the necessity of a shock. Until we accomplish this greater understanding, we might consider the possibility that alleviation of the shock, in whatever form it may take, may serve to stabilize an old pattern and deter movement to a new, higher level patterning. The fluctuating patterns of harmony-disharmony can be regarded as peaks and troughs of the rhythmic life process. Most of us prefer harmony, but we may need the repatterning that disharmony can stimulate.

The cyclic stages of growth, as defined by Ainsworth-Land (1982), may help to explain the process. Each stage of growth is associated with different feelings. In the first, formative stage, one feels good when one can control other people and things, as in the child learning to control his or her body and the mother controlling the child. As one moves into the normative second stage of growth, the good feelings are associated with exerting influence over others, with persuading others to think as we do and to act in accordance with our wishes. In the third stage, mutuality, feeling good is associated with sharing—the giving up and taking in of making and breaking bonds. Then a shift occurs. In the transformation that takes place in the fourth stage, *the old rules no longer apply*. Feeling good is no longer the necessary concomitant of growth. One experiences the disconnectedness that is associated with pain (or perhaps disease). Things seem to be falling apart. This is the disorder, or disequilibrium, that is the necessary predecessor of a new order, or higher level of consciousness. There is a tendency to want to hold on to the old rules, but the need is to let go into a new realm. We need to be able to tolerate the uncertainty and ambiguity that precedes the clarity of the evolving pattern.

It is possible to move to higher levels of consciousness without the necessity of disease. The degree of fluidity with which we interact with stress determines how disabling it will be (Bentov, 1978; Moss, 1981). Openness allows the energies to pass through. This means that we accept the experience as *our* experience regardless of how contrary it is to what we might have wished would happen. If we reject the experience, we reject ourselves and we initiate the process of defending ourselves against ourself (fighting off the offender), and so stress-related physical changes occur. When we let go of personal control (which we don't have anyway), life is de-stressed. This does not mean that we do not act or that we passively are run over by whatever comes our way. It simply means we accept it and interact with it as *our* experience. We recognize that we are one aspect of a much larger whole that is evolving to a higher order, and we learn from the experience. Moss (1981) believes "that all disease and all suffering starts as we begin to recoil away from this deeper intuition of the vastness and indefinable eternity of Self. When the fear or doubt arises, which it does over and over again, it becomes a signal that it is time to let go, rebalance and find an unconditional allowing of life" (p. 29).

PATTERNS OF ENERGY EXCHANGE

The pattern being signaled by the disease can be seen and understood in terms of the energy exchange of person-environment interaction. Physical illness or intense emotional activity may be regarded as manifestations of blocked energy beyond our awareness (Moss, 1981). Although we cannot always "see" energy exchange, we accept that it is a characteristic of the human field (e.g. the energy patterns depicted by a electrocardiogram or electroencephalogram). Disease makes it possible for us to envision a *total* pattern of the energy field of a person. For example, hypertension may connote a pattern of contained energy, hyperthyroidism a pattern of diffuse, multidirectional energy, or diabetes the inability to use available energy. Each of these patterns varies, of course, according to the unique configuration of each person-environment situation.

The disease can be regarded as a clue to pattern and can assist people in becoming aware of their pattern of interacting with the environment. A number of years ago a friend of mine had a full-blown case of hyperthyroidism and was being treated by a leading endocrinologist in New York City. She had been taking medication for approximately a year with very little progress in eliminating her symptoms. The endocrinologist had indicated that she probably would have to have surgery to remove the gland. But before she pursued that alternative she went to see Dora Kunz, a sensitive person who has the ability to see the patterns of people's interactions as they relate to their diseases (Weber, 1984). My friend related the things Dora told her in her interview, and this is what I gleaned from it: Dora could "see" that my friend's energy was being diffused in every direction (in a slightly diminished intensity, probably because of the medications she was taking) and that it was not relevant to tell my friend to curtail her activities in order to channel her energy better. The pattern of intense multidirectional energy expenditure was her way of life. The only thing Dora could suggest was that my friend make sure she took in enough energy to sustain her way of life.

To fill in some background, my friend was the oldest of nine children and was looked to for advice and assistance not only by her siblings but also by her parents. She was a member of a religious community of nuns and freely fulfilled her responsibilities to other members of the community on their frequent visits to or through New York. She was a faculty member in a large urban university and enthusiastically carried more than her share of teaching responsibilities along with a larger-than-usual number of committee responsibilities. She could rarely say "no" to any request. She was a caring friend to many people, typically staying up half the night to bake a birthday cake or perform some similar favor.

Dora's picture of her energy going in many directions was true to her life. And it was accurate that she was not taking in enough energy to sustain that way of life—not taking time to sleep or eat or rest. When I really began to think about it, her thyroid gland was trying to produce the energy she needed. The medical/surgical approach to diminish or delete the activity of the thyroid gland was just the opposite of what her system was trying to accomplish.

My friend did begin to pay more attention to her energy intake. She did not have to have surgery and was even able to eliminate or greatly reduce the medications she was taking. I do not want to imply that simply balancing her energy intake-output did the trick. I surmise that the transforming factor was the *insight* she gained regarding her own pattern of life, the understanding that Young (1976b) refers to as accelerating the evolution of consciousness. Perhaps, as has already been suggested, she discovered herself in this pattern, found peace in the congruity, and was able to move to a higher level of organization and harmony. Moss (1981) states:

> We must attain higher energy states to begin to transmute the reality that appears unchangeable at our present energy level. Whether this occurs through the spontaneous awakening of energies or through a disease process is of little importance. (p. 101)

The pattern of a person that eventually manifests itself as disease is primary. The disease is a manifestation of the underlying pattern of energy exchange. This point is germane to Chinese medicine (Tiller, 1973) and has been illustrated in plants by Kirlian photography (Ostrander & Schroeder, 1971). Ravitz's early work correlating bioelectrical potentials with disease indicated that the change in the bioelectrical field preceded subjective and behavioral changes associated with illness (Ravitz, 1962).

The literature is replete with examples of personality patterns that correlate with disease states. The patterns associated with cancer and with heart disease are probably the most widely acknowledged. LeShan (1966) described the cancer patient as having a life history pattern of despair characterized by denial and repression. The pattern typically includes a childhood of isolation, hopelessness, and despair, following in adulthood by the establishment of a meaningful, satisfying relationship that is subsequently lost, with accompanying despair (LeShan, 1966; Schmale & Iker, 1966). The individual is marked by feelings of isolation, neglect, and despair but is unable to communicate the hurt, anger, or hostility that is felt (Abse et al., 1974; LeShan, 1977; Nemeth & Meezi, 1967; Pollard, 1981). Diminished immune reaction that often occurs in response to severe loss, sadness, and despair (Bathrop, 1977; Pelletier, 1977; Selye, 1956) completes the picture of the pattern of person with cancer: a lifetime of despair and repression, together with a diminished immune system and significant personal loss.

Type A persons, those thought to be prone to heart disease, have been described as aggressive, impatient, and involved in an "incessant struggle to achieve more and more in less and less time" (Friedman & Rosenman, 1974). The propensity to display hostility in explosive vocal mannerisms has been pinpointed as an important indicator of heart disease (Matthews et al., cited in Dembroski et al., 1984). Previous research revealing increased levels of physiological parameters of stress in Type A individuals led Dembroski et al. to characterize Type A persons as "hot reactors," i.e., persons who have stronger physiological reactions to stress than their Type B counterparts.

Although I cite these profiles to illustrate a point, I do so with caution because of my conviction that it is essential to consider the *unique* pattern of each person-environment interaction. Even though two persons may have the same disease, the complex configuration of their pattern of interaction is very different. The profiles describing cancer and heart disease patients should be studied from the standpoint of patterns of energy exchange within the person-family-community field of interaction. For example, one might speculate from the foregoing descriptions that the pattern of people with cancer is one of low, depleted energy manifesting itself in low ability to "fight back" either verbally or in relation to proliferating cells, whereas the person with heart disease manifests a pattern of high energy that "bursts out" in explosive verbal attacks and myocardial infarctions.

DISEASE AS INTEGRATING FACTOR

It seems strange to say (strange because it is part of the revolutionary shift) but disease may be the only way a person can get in touch with his or her pattern. Many of us have lived our lives in such a way that we have not become fully aware of ourselves or our own pattern. The pattern may then manifest itself in a more "unconscious" manner, in terms of changes that may be interpreted as maladaptive, or disease, but which may represent movement to a higher level of consciousness. For instance, certain forms of psychosis may be an indication of a person's involvement in an important personal transformation (Pelletier, 1978). Physical disease may serve the same purpose— even more so—since physical changes associated with internalization of stress may represent a person's inability to be fully aware of stress. Moss (1981) relates that "what may unfold unconsciously at one level of consciousness and finally present as disease may now be perceived as an energetic shift which becomes an unfolding process" (p. 75). This relates to Moss's position that some of what is labeled disease might be considered stalled or overly rapid penetrations of higher energies. And this is similar to Rogers' (1970) position that some of our diseases are manifestations of evolutionary emergence of higher energy states. According to Moss, our individual behaviors (diseases?) describe not who we are but "what we don't dissolve into" (how we separate ourselves). It takes energy to maintain the me that is separate, and this may translate into disease.

Disease may be considered an integrating factor (Stone, 1978) and, as such, is important in the evolutionary development of the person. Evolution thrives on tension (Watson, 1978). Contrary to what one might think, disequilibrium is important in maintaining active exchange with the environment (Jantsch, 1980), and active exchange with the environment is essential for growth (Land, 1973). The tension characteristic of disease may provide an important disequilibriant in the growth process and therefore may be regarded as a facilitator of that process. We evolve by having our own equilibrium thrown off balance and then discovering how to attain a new state of balance, temporarily, and then move on to another phase of disequilibrium. This is a natural process, according to Fuller (1975): "The forces of the field of energy . . . interoscillate through the symmetry of equilibrium to various asymmetries, never pausing at equilibrium. The vector equilibrium itself is only a referential pattern of conceptual relationships at which nature never pauses" (p. 27). Dossey (1982) agrees and views disease as a natural perturbation that offers human beings the chance to evolve to a new and higher level of complexity.

Disease can help people see themselves and their interaction with others more clearly. The following example illustrates how disease was a transforming process for an entire family. A man in South Dakota shared this experience with me:

My father's bout with amyotrophic lateral sclerosis is a very inspirational story. He had been studied as a polio victim at age 11. Massive surgery left him with a pronounced hunchback and limp with very little use of his left arm.

His life was a series of tenacious episodes with "overcoming"; generally by gritting his teeth and saying sonofabitch he was able to "muscle" and aggressively overcome most obstacles. He taught himself how to bowl, drive, golf, and, more importantly, deal with people who could not deal with his appearance and disability. His eight years in the State House as our county representative were testimony to his perseverance over polio and his disfigurement. His successful business career and work in Rotary and JCs were memorable.

ALS was diagnosed in 1966. The physicians who did workups on him differed about his polio and his ALS. They concurred that life expectancy would be approximately two years. Six years after that . . . and a remarkable story, he died.

His first assessment leading to ALS was a weakening in his golf grip, then a tiring at work. His compensation was consistent: Get tough! Fight it! Then one physician said it was likely muscle weakening from his earlier surgery and atrophy from polio as a child, and he tried more reasonable accommodation by taking naps. This was the first of what I would call "consciousness expansion" . . . I began to see him, as more accepting of his abilities . . . not just his disabilities.

The next six years were a monument to adaptation, personal awareness, and heightened communication: fluid intake, calorie intake, stress awareness, many visits with physicians and researchers, medications, bladder infections and pneumonia . . . and two trips to the emergency room with prolonged hospitalization.

Throughout it all was a remarkable woman who helped this process—both from her selfish point of view and from his. How can we deal with this pain, that slurring of speech, this feeling of frustration about family and friends? How can we deal with your death, this hospitalization, these insensitive hospital staff, and with the family who loves you but feels as helpless as you? Mom was phenomenal.

I saw Dad go from an aggressive, seemingly insensitive man to an accepting, aware, and tender person. Imagine giving this kind of father a bath and washing his testicles. Imagine giving this kind of man his meals through a straw. Imagine communicating with a politician and insurance salesman who can no longer talk. He did and we did . . . but mostly because he let us and helped us.

There were times when his expanding consciousness did some pretty direct reversions!* Trying to get residents to treat him with dignity, nurses to be patient in understanding him, and friends to not be afraid to come visit him. He would blow his stack . . . and cry . . . and we would all weep for him, his dignity, and his very lonely struggle.

Part of his expanding consciousness (and that of the family) was the excitement and partial ownership he felt in my mother's expanding role and consciousness as a business woman. In three short years she took over the agency, passed each and every state exam and license, and was elected Businesswoman of the Year. You think he didn't play a part in that? What pride he took as she studied for her tests by his bedside, as he helped her understand the business and the agency.

Four years' of "This may be Dad's last holiday" put tremendous pressures on the entire family—those of us away in college, those still home. Mom and Dad traveled extensively, visited us, and said "goodbye" to us many times.

We can see from this example that we are not separate people with separate diseases. We are open energy systems constantly interacting and evolving with each other. The pattern manifested by a disease does not stop with one person but is part of the greater whole. Basic to this view is the premise of the undivided wholeness of the universe (Bohm, 1980). In the process of considering the pattern of interaction of an individual with the environment, one inevitably considers the pattern of interaction of the family.

FAMILY AND COMMUNITY PATTERNS

The premise that illness in one family member may be a function of the pattern of family interaction was introduced in the fifties in psychiatry in relation to the schizophrenogenic family and has been extended to other diagnoses, including

---

*My position on this is that there are no reversions. Expressing anger and/or sadness would be an expression of his expanding consciousness.

anorexia nervosa and diabetes (Minuchin, et al., 1978). The premise that disease is a manifestation of the pattern of the family can be applied to any type of family situation: the family in which a parent has a degenerative disease or a myocardial infarction, the family in which a child has a developmental disability, the family in which an elderly parent faces many of the pathologies associated with aging, and so on.

There is no intent here to imply causality. The pattern simply *is*. The disease simply is a manifestation of the pattern, a pattern of evolving consciousness of the family. Central to this view is the premise that disease is an integrative and transformative factor in the family system. If a family member's becoming "ill" is the only way the family can become conscious of itself as a unit and of each other and their interactions with the environment, then that is health in process for that family. The previous example illustrates disease as an integrative factor in a family's evolving consciousness.

A crisis with its attendant increase in intensity of family relationships facilitates change in the family system. The crisis, such as the illness in the father in the previous example, stimulates a fundamental revision of a family's shared pattern of perceiving each other. The new reality becomes the point around which the family organizes. The family who thrives in the process of crisis often develops an entirely new sense of its own potency. A new pattern born in crisis serves as an orienting perspective to family strategizing in daily life (Reiss & Oliveri, 1980).

Viewing the individual as an open system in the context of the family as an open system leads to the consideration of interaction with the community. Here too the previous assumptions apply. Health of the community is conceptualized in terms of changing patterns of energy exchange in the evolution of the system. The pattern of disease endemic to a community can be considered a manifestation of the pattern of community health. The diversity and quality of interaction within the community and between the community and its larger environment are indicators of the level of consciousness, and thus of the health, of the community.

• • •

The process of life is toward higher levels of consciousness. Sometimes this process is smooth, pleasant, harmonious; other times it is difficult and disharmonious, as in disease. Moss (1981) writes:

> I believe that, when the new level of energy is attained, the forces that might have configured disease at the old level no longer need operate. If it is not attained, then the disease probably perseveres and physical death may become the transformative door. In either case, transformation of consciousness has occurred, and to a deeper level of our Beingness this may be all that really matters. (p. 101)

The conclusions of Lerner and Remen (1985), based on their work with cancer patients, support this view:

> But what is most striking to me about many of these people with cancer has nothing to do with evidence of extended disease-free intervals or life expectancy. What amazes and touches me is that through this difficult life passage they have found inner resources of strength, wisdom, and insight that they often had not experienced before. They do not live with certainties of clear victories. They live with the knowledge that the cancer process may worsen or return at any time, and with the personal conviction that how they live may affect when or whether it does so. But the kind of life they develop is also the one that they would want to follow even if their efforts had no impact on the course of the disease. (p. 32)

When we begin to think of ourselves as centers of energy within an overall pattern of expanding consciousness, we can begin to see that what we sense of our lives is part of a much larger whole. First the pattern of consciousness that is the person interacts within the pattern of consciousness that is the family and physical surroundings and within the pattern that is the person's larger environmental affiliations, such as work or school, and then within the pattern of the local community, and continuing on within the pattern of the universe.

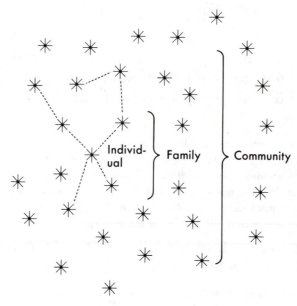

Fig. 4 The Individual, Family and Community as Centers of Consciousness

CHAPTER 3

THE PATTERN OF

EXPANDING CONSCIOUSNESS

What we are concerned with is the health of persons in interaction with the environment. The total pattern of person-environment can be viewed as a network of consciousness. The assumption is made that consciousness is coextensive in the universe and resides in all matter (Bentov, 1978; Muses, 1978). Persons as individuals, and human beings as a species, are identified by their patterns of consciousness. The person does not *possess* consciousness—the person *is* consciousness.

The key to understanding this view of consciousness is in its definition. Consciousness is defined as the informational capacity of the system: the capacity of the system to interact with its environment. In the human system the informational capacity includes all of our present and developing knowledge about the nervous system, the endocrine system, the immune system, the genetic code, and so on. Knowledge of these and other systems reveals the complexity of the human system and how the information of the system determines a person's response to the environment. The immune system is a good example. It is set up in such a way that when foreign particles enter the system, it produces other particles designed to combat the foreign invaders. This kind of information then is part of the consciousness of the system. The more highly developed the system, the more complex the informational capacity, and the more varied and more numerous the responses to the environment.

Consciousness can be seen in the quantity and quality of this interaction. Jantsch (1980) points out that "If consciousness is defined as the degree of autonomy a system gains in the dynamic relations with its environment, even the simplest autopoietic systems . . . have a primitive form of *consciousness*" (p. 40). As the quantity of consciousness increases, the more numerous and more varied are the responses to the environment. As the quality of consciousness increases, there is a higher frequency of response, such as increased agility or speed of response. In terms of human interaction, an individual at higher levels of consciousness has a greater repertoire of responses to any given situation and does so with ease and speed. There is a greater refinement of response in terms of insight, context, and detail (Bentov, 1978).

The evolution of consciousness is illustrated in Fig. 5. The range is from "inanimate" objects (like rocks) at the bottom of the graph to astral and spiritual "beings" above the human level. Rocks display a low level of consciousness in terms of quantity and quality of interaction with the environment; yet there *is* some interaction, and when one considers the interactional capacity of some crystals, it may be that the consciousness of rocks is much greater than we have imagined (as fans of Johnny Hart's *B.C.* are well aware).

Moving up the vertical axis of the graph to plants, animals, and eventually human beings, one can see the increasing complexity of the categories with the concomitant increasing ability to interact with the environment based on the information of the system, e.g., the ability of plants to extract and utilize nutrients from the environment, the mobility of animals, the

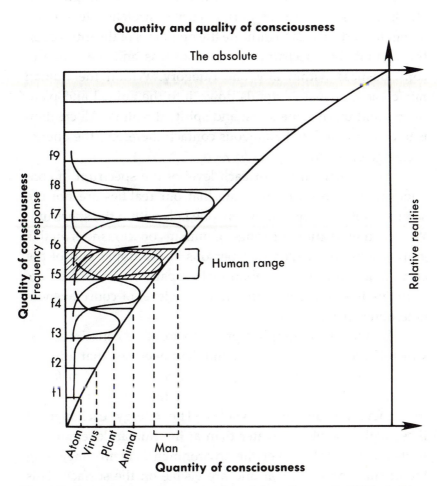

Fig. 5 Evolution of Consciousness. Adapted from Benton, I. (1978). *Stalking the wild pendulum*. New York: E.P. Dutton, p. 60.

higher cortical abilities of humans. With increases in levels of consciousness, the system forms more intricate nervous systems, capable of interacting with nature in more complex patterns. Bentov (1978) uses normal curves stretched to infinity along the vertical axis to indicate the openness of the interaction throughout the spectrum of consciousness and the range of consciousness within any one category. Within the human range consciousness extends down into the animal and plant ranges and up into the astral and spiritual realms. All creation is in constant and instantaneous contact; therefore, the energy exchange curve never goes to zero.

The normal curves for each level of the spectrum of consciousness are used to illustrate that our realities are not the same. Reality depends on where one falls within the spectrum. When contemplating the range of human consciousness on this graph, one can imagine that persons at the upper end of the curve might appear to be abnormal (or pathological?) to others in the middle of the human range. The level of consciousness determines reality.

The top of the graph represents absolute consciousness, which Bentov compares to a boundless deep sea that appears calm and smooth *but contains tremendous energy and is full of creative potential*. It consists of infinitely fine vibration of high-frequency, low-amplitude waves. The energy exchange at these higher levels is greater than at the human level and affords greater control over the environment. Again, imagining the ocean, ripples appear and are visible on the surface. This is our manifest, physical reality. Matter *is* the vibrating, changing component of pure consciousness (Bentov, 1978). These descriptions by Bentov correspond to Bohm's analogies of the implicate/explicate order. The calm, unruffled sea of creative potential corresponds to the implicate order; the waves of matter correspond to the explicate order. Bentov main-

tains that all matter is evolving toward higher levels of consciousness.

This view of matter as the manifestation of consciousness
reaffirms the unitary nature of mind-body. Mind and matter
are made of the same basic stuff. The difference is in the speed
and intensity of the energy waves. Mind represents faster,
higher energy waves, and matter represents slower, lower energy waves. Bentov offers the analogy of ice and steam: One
is solid, the other more diffuse, but both are manifestations of
water in different form.

The high-frequency, high-energy waves have a low am-
plitude. As they approach infinity, they approach a straight line
of absolute consciousness:

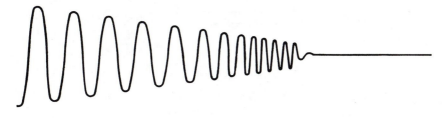

Fig. 6

"Absolute consciousness is a state in which contrasting concepts become reconciled and fused. Movement and rest fuse
into one" (Bentov, 1978).

THE EVOLUTION OF NEW FORMS

The creative potential embedded in absolute consciousness, or the implicate order, has a self-organizing capability.
The process of evolving to higher levels of consciousness is
consistent with Rogers' (1970) assumption of increasing com-

plexity in living systems and is supported by Prigogine's theory of dissipative structures.*

Dissipative structures have two complementary aspects: (1) deterministic behavior based on the average values of the variables involved and (2) amplification of the fluctuations of the system leading to a change in structure. A new order appears when a giant fluctuation becomes stabilized by exchange of energy with the environment. Prigogine illustrates this process as follows:

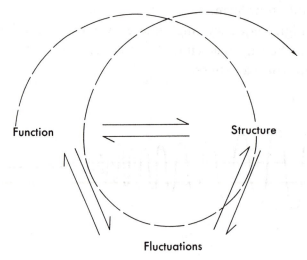

Fig. 7 Prigogine's Process of Dissipative Structures

---

*This theory explains the paradox of decreasing order (entropy) in physical processes and increasing order (negative entropy) in living systems (Prigogine, 1980; Prigogine et al., 1977). Entropy is based on observations within a closed system (linear transformations close to equilibirum), one in which energy can enter and leave but mass cannot. Such a system will evolve through irreversible processes to a state of maximum entropy, i.e., maximum disorder. This type of evolution is not the basis for the evolution of living systems. Living systems are open systems, systems undergoing irreversible nonlinear transformation far from equilibrium. These systems are capable of exchanging both energy and matter with the environment. When properties of thermodynamics are extended to open systems, new properties emerge: the capacity for self-organi-

Continued on p. 39.

The function component represents the stable, deterministic force; the fluctuations represent the chance element, such as critical events, and yield changes in the physical world in the form of mutants or in the social world in the form of behavioral and technological change. This evolution requires energy from the environment. A single form of species "in competition for resources evolves in such a way that hitherto untapped resources are exploited, and each resource is exploited with increasing effectiveness" (Prigogine et al., 1977, p. 3).

The similarities between the functioning of a society and that of dissipative structures are described as follows:

> Firstly, societies have complex non-linear interactions between their elements derived from the cooperation and conflicts involved in the attempts of individuals and groups to attain "goals." Secondly, they are subject to local "behavioral fluctuations," meaning that sometimes new behavior can appear, such as an invention, a modification of group organization, or a new goal or belief, and this can either be suppressed by the social environment or will grow and spread until the society itself is modified. Here again we find the dual aspects of change and determinism, and the theory briefly described here . . . serve as a background for discussion of the evolution of social systems." (Prigogine et al., 1977, p. 4)

In comparing this theory to their observations of planetary motion, these authors comment: "Instead of finding stability and harmony, wherever we look we discover evolutionary pro-

---

zation, spontaneous shift from lower to higher level of organization complexity (Prigogine et al., 1977). A major point is that irreversible processes play a fundamental constructive role.

A local region of the living system (e.g., an individual human system, a family system, or a community system) is both a positive-entropy (disorder) source that dumps into the environment and a negative-entropy (order) sink which drains negative entropy from the environment so as to increase the internal order and complexity of the local region. Prigogine names such self-organizing systems "dissipative structures," since they maintain their organizational complexity by continually dissipating high entropy energy that they produce back into the environment.

cesses leading to diversification and increasing complexity" (pp. 5–6).

Prigogine's theory is based on the fact that all dynamic systems fluctuate, but rather than averaging out, the process itself becomes supraordinate to the random perturbations and shifts to *a new, higher order*, more complex structural form. At this new level of organization, a new set of functional principles applies. A new order is attained through fluctuation. The richer the resources of the environment, the greater the diversity. The more elements that enter into interaction, the greater the chance of instability and, therefore, the greater the chance of new traits coming into being (Prigogine et al., 1977).

Sheldrake (1983) also addresses the phenomenon of new forms coming into being. In his hypothesis of formative causation, he states that characteristic forms and behavior of physical, chemical, and biological systems in the present moment are determined by invisible organizing fields acting across time and space. He refers to these fields as morphogenetic fields, which he conceives as being without mass or energy.

Sheldrake cites a 1920 learning experiment on rats conducted by William McDougall. In these experiments, the task remained the same but later generations of rats learned the task more quickly than earlier generations. In subsequent experiments designed to replicate this finding, the first generation learned almost as quickly as McDougall's last generation; some learned immediately without error. Sheldrake hypothesizes that the first generation established a morphogenetic field for the specific behavior being learned and that this field guided the behavior of other generations via morphic resonance.

According to Sheldrake, the effect of the morphogenetic field is not diminished by space or time and is cumulative. This theory lends an explanation to the observed phenomenon that the difficulty of synthesizing new compounds becomes increasingly easier once the compound has been formed the first time, and this facility is apparent in laboratories great distances from each other. *It gives pattern a role in the development and evolution* of *physical and biological systems.* The activity of the central nervous system can be understood in terms of spatiotemporal patterns of chemical and electrical activity (energy) or as patterns of consciousness.

Whyte (1974), in his final philosophical treatise, speaks of the two great general tendencies of order and disorder and points out the fallacy of their *apparent* opposition. Rather he sees them as complementary and indispensable antagonists. He speaks of these tendencies as contrasting coexisting systems, not the clash of opposed principles. Watson (1978) speculates that evolution requires a rival plan, that DNA is joined by a rival program in the mitochondria, that sets evolution free from the constraints of the body, from the dictates of the genes. Evolution thrives on instability and tension.

PATTERN RECOGNITION AS TURNING POINT IN THE EVOLUTION OF CONSCIOUSNESS

Young (1976b) identifies three types of evolution. The first involves the genotype, changes effected by DNA in the design of the mechanism. The second manifests itself as animal instinct, or learned behavior, and begins only when there is the possibility of choice. The third, incorporating the previous two, is possible for human beings; it is the possibility of *understanding* and brings with it much more rapid evolutionary change. This type of evolution is not gradual, as are the previous types, but occurs instantaneously: "Primarily it is *recognition*, recognition of a principle, realization of a truth, reconciliation of a duality, *satori*. It is at once the privilege of man, and the formative principle that enables man to evolve" (p. 180). Insight has been equated with pattern recognition (Hart, 1978) and with the inner voice that some people consider their intuition. Pattern recognition is the key to human evolution.

Young (1976b) takes the position that the evolution of matter represents a fall from total freedom into determinism. From Young's perspective, the stage of determinate matter represents a turning point at which matter takes on one of the characteristics of living systems and is able to utilize energy from the environment in a self-organizing fashion, i.e., the reversal of entropy. He sees action rather than matter as basic:

> . . . it is no longer appropriate to think of the universe as a gradually subsiding agitation of billiard balls. The universe, far from being a desert of inert particles, is a theatre of increasingly complex organization, a stage for development in which man has a definite place, and without any upper limit to his evolution. (p. xxiv)

Young designates light as the whole from which the universe has evolved and as the origin of everything, including "the eternal now of consciousness" (p. 28). Movement from light to determinate matter involves increasing loss of freedom, or increase in constraints; movement from determinate matter back to the light incorporates corresponding gains in freedom.

Wilbur (1979) sees the emergence of the human being's consciousness as separate from the world as a stage of development in which duality exists. The meaning of the developmental process is the transcendence of the separate self into superconsciousness, a return to the wholeness of the absolute, and with it the end of the tyranny of time.

The testimony of these scientists/philosophers presents some agreement that life is evolving in the direction of increasing complexity toward higher levels of consciousness, that complementary forces of order and disorder maintain a fluctuating field that periodically transcends itself and shifts into a higher order of functioning, and that in humans this evolutionary process is facilitated by insight and means a transcendence of the spatial-temporal self. Some would argue that consciousness is primary to matter, that thought precedes form. However, it is probably more accurate to say that consciousness is not separate from matter, that there is a common ground for both.

HEALTH AS THE EVOLUTION OF CONSCIOUSNESS

The process of the evolution of consciousness is also the process of health. The human being comes from a state of potential consciousness into the world of determinate matter and has the capacity for understanding that will enable him or her to gain insight regarding his/her pattern. This instantaneous insight represents a turning point in evolving consciousness with concomitant gains in freedom. Young (1976b) regards the stage of determinate matter as a necessary laboratory for testing one's understanding of the way things work. He sees the life process as a sequence of learning to *use* a "law" rather than be blocked by it.

This task is one that I see as particularly relevant where disease is concerned. The physical manifestations of disease may be considered evidence of how one is interacting with the environment. In this sense this illustrates the laboratory to which Young refers. The task is to gain an understanding of that pattern and try to work with it.

The central theme of Young's theory is that a self, or a universe, is of the same nature. The essential nature is undefinable, but the beginning and the end are characterized by complete freedom, unrestricted choice. The steps in between are a sequence of, first, losses of freedom, as identity in the form of a physical being evolves, and then a reversal of these losses as entropy is reversed and understanding evolves.

There is a corollary between my model of health as expanding consciousness and Young's conception of the evolution of human beings. Young (1976b) describes this development as first a loss of freedom and then a reversal of the process as the human being moves toward total freedom:

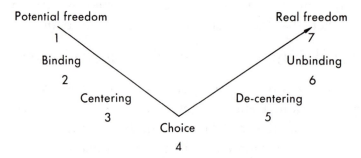

Fig. 8 Young's Theory of Human Evolution

The goal, according to Young, is to reach a higher level of development, and the process is one of interaction of persons with one another and with the social state.

The second stage of Young's model is characterized by binding. The individual is sacrificed for the sake of the collective. Everything is regulated for the individual, and there is no need for initiative. In the third stage, centering, an individual identity is established and along with it self-consciousness and self-determination. Individualism emerges in the self's break with authority. The fourth stage, choice, is the turning point. The task of the fourth stage is to learn the "law." The emphasis is on science and on searching for laws. It involves a more advanced stage of combination of people and things and an eventual realization that the devices invented are no longer solutions to the situation. Answers to the problems require a different kind of solution from those previously considered "progress." A new awareness of self-limitation precedes inner growth. The turning point is a kind of inward, self-generated reformation.

The fifth stage, decentering, begins when the "law" is

learned. In this stage emphasis shifts from the development of self (individuation) to dedication to something greater than the individual self. The person experiences outstanding competence; works have a life of their own beyond the creator. The task is the transcendance of the ego. Form is transcended, and energy becomes the dominant feature in terms of animation, vitality, a quality that is somehow infinite. Pattern is higher than form, and so the pattern can manifest itself in different forms. In this stage the person experiences the power of unlimited growth and has learned how to build order against the trend of disorder. The reversal of entropy, however, is destructive to the system unless the energy gained is used to produce other systems. The morality of the fifth stage is the "relinquishing of the power" but not of the products of this power. Young (1976b) explains, "There will come a time *in the lives of each of us* when we will go on or be destroyed, but this time will not come until we wield so much power that the misuse of it would destroy ourselves" (p. 216).

We don't really know what happens at the sixth stage and beyond because these stages are not physical. We have some glimpse of the superhuman powers that exist by examining the events in the lives of those known to be evolved to higher states: healings, appearances in different forms, etc.

Corollaries to these stages from my model are:

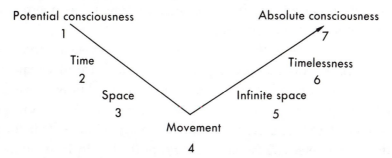

Fig. 9 Young's Process Applied to Expanding Consciousness

We come into being from a state of potential consciousness, are bound in time, find our identity in space, and through movement learn the "law" of the way things work and make choices that ultimately take us beyond space and time to a state of absolute consciousness.

Early in the development of my theory I was dealing primarily with the loss of freedom occurring in the second, third, and fourth substages of the process. Development of the physical self is necessarily binding in time and space. Movement provides a way of controlling one's environment. As physical disability brings about restriction in body movement, these losses of freedom become even more apparent. The restrictions in movement-space-time force an awareness that extends beyond the physical self. This awareness corresponds, I think, to the inward, self-generated reformation that Young speaks of as the turning point of the process. It comes about when the things that have worked for us in the past no longer work. We have to seek answers that are different from what we have previously considered "progress." The new awareness comes from a limitation of self that at the same time becomes a process of inner growth, a transformation.

The next stage is the throwing off of centeredness or concerns with one's own self, one's own boundaries, or space. It is recognition that one's essence extends beyond the physical boundaries and is in effect "boundarylessness," as one moves to higher levels of consciousness.

Progression to the sixth stage involves increasing freedom from time. This may be experienced in a sense of expanded time, a dilatation of a moment of time as we know it. Young (1976a) speculates that the reversal of time as we know it might be considered an inverse of time. If "normal" time (T) is long, then the inverse (1/T) would be very short: eternity in an instant.

He adds that in a photon, energy is inversely proportional to time and implies that in an "anti" world, there might be unlimited energy in an instant of time. The experience of expanded time is one of going more deeply into the present and having the experience of all time.

The last stage is absolute consciousness, which has been equated with love. In this state all opposites are reconciled. This kind of love embraces all experience equally and unconditionally: pain as well as pleasure, failure as well as success, ugliness as well as beauty, disease as well as non-disease. The process of learning the "law," reversing entropy, and moving toward higher levels of consciousness may appear as quanta of action, each at higher levels of interaction.

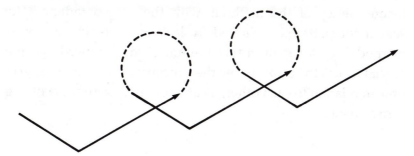

Fig. 10 Critical Choices Leading to Higher Levels of Consciousness

CHAPTER 4

TIME-SPACE-MOVEMENT AS

MANIFESTATIONS OF CONSCIOUSNESS

Operationalization of this model of health as expanding consciousness has been approached in two ways: (1) by research methods designed to describe and test the relationships between the major concepts—movement, time, space, and consciousness—and (2) by attempts to describe evolving patterns of consciousness in terms of the integration of movement-space-time. Findings based on traditional research are limited by the incongruency of the methods with the new paradigm. The search for patterns is limited by lack of a clearly developed methodology for pattern recognition. I am convinced that the crucial task is to be able to see the concepts of movement-space-time in relation to each other, all at once, as patterns of evolving consciousness.

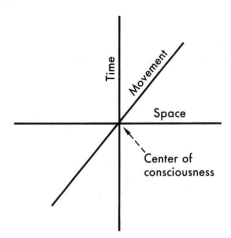

Fig. 11 Persons as Centers of Consciousness with Movement-Time-Space Configurations

The intersection of movement-space-time represents the person as a center of consciousness and varies from person to person, place to place, and time to time.

Some of the findings arrived at by both approaches are presented here to illustrate the relevancy of this conceptual model to current health care situations. The order in which they are presented corresponds to the evolutionary process adapted from Young (1976b): binding in time and space, integration through movement, and transformation beyond space-time to the highest level of consciousness.

TIME AND TIMING

The rhythm of biological phenomena is a vivid portrayal of the embeddedness of matter (consciousness) in space-time. Twenty years ago Stephens (1965) challenged nursing to consider the relevance of temporal patterns in patient care. She described some of the rhythmic phenomena in human beings and animals and the possible hazards of drug and radiation therapy if the varying susceptibility of the organism during the 24-hour daily cycle is not taken into consideration. Data were available, for instance, on a drug that has a fatal effect at one point within the circadian cycle and a therapeutic effect at another point. She suggested that more attention be given to the rhythms of people and the effects of the demands of the "therapeutic" regimen, particularly within the hospital situation.

Now, twenty years later, there is some indication that consideration is being given to the varying therapeutic effectiveness of specific treatments at different times of day and to the timeliness of teaching efforts in relation to the readiness of the patient. However the question remains as to what extent the individual rhythms of patients are being recognized and honored in the planning of their care.

Take, for instance, the pattern of sleep-wakefulness. Individual patterns of sleep-wakefulness differ considerably. These differences are somehow related to body temperature, and body temperature fluctuations appear to differ from person to person.

The sleep-wake cycle, if allowed to fluctuate without any external controls, will assume a circadian cycle of approximately 25 ± 0.5 hours (Minors & Waterhouse, 1984). The waking of the individual then moves forward a little each day in relation to light-dark fluctuation of the 24-hour period until at one point a new synchronization of the sleep-wake and light-dark cycles is established. During the period when individuals are out of phase with the external demands of the 24-hour period, they may experience diminished alertness and efficiency and feel as though they are having an "off" day—which indeed they are. In addition, the sleep-wake cycle is closely associated with the function of the adrenal gland. The peak output of adrenal corticosteroids occurs just prior to waking. The level of output remains high during the waking hours and steadily declines to its lowest level of output during the sleep period. The trough of the adrenal output occurs at a time when the steroids are least needed. Consider, however, what this normal fluctuation means in relation to the demands of early morning surgery or same day surgery.

Correlated with the temperature rhythm is the productivity of the individual; persons are most productive and most accurate in their productivity at the peak of the temperature rhythm (Colquhoun, 1971; Kleitman, 1963). Time of day also appears to be a factor in how persons with different personality types perform. Blake (1967) found introverts to be more efficient in the morning, whereas extroverts are at their peak in the afternoon. These differences in alertness and productivity are relevant considerations when patients are engaged in learning new tasks. Rodgers (1972) found that both introverts and extroverts preferred more personal space in the morning than in the afternoon, a finding with implications for the personal care administered to patients by nurses.

An interesting experiment conducted by a nurse in an intensive care unit revealed significantly less depression in patients who were given more control over their environment in terms of the timing of their daily bath, timing of their visitors, and arrangement of their greeting cards within their own allotted space (Kallio, 1979). When the experiment ended, however, these freedoms in terms of time and space were not maintained.*

Time perception, or the subjective sense of passing time, has been shown to vary with time of day and is thought to be synchronized with other circadian rhythms, particularly body temperature (Pfaff, 1968; Siffre, 1964; Stephens, 1965). An increase in body temperature is related to the subjective sense of a greater amount of time passing than is revealed by clock time and thus the feeling that time is dragging. The opposite is true for a decrease in body temperature. This means that the sense of time varies from individual to individual in relation to temperature cycle and also, more markedly, in instances of abnormal temperature elevation.

Individuals may not be particularly aware of the fluctuations described and may become upset when other persons' sense of time is different from their own. Kaufman (1969) pointed this out many years ago and suggested that the incongruity of different experiences of time might produce additional stress for patients if not adequately understood and addressed by the nurse.

---

*M. Mirr, personal communication, May 1, 1985.

Cultural differences in the time experience are among the most subtle and at the same time most frustrating. Hall's characterization of temporal patterns as monochronic or polychronic illustrates the incongruities and resultant stress encountered when people from different time patterns interact (Hall, 1959, 1984).

Monochronic time, characteristic of the American-European culture, is linear and compartmentalized. It is related to industrialization and scheduling and is arbitrary and imposed. It is oriented to task or procedures rather than to people and, like money, can be saved and spent within this context. Polychronic time, on the contrary, stresses involvement with people and completion of transactions rather than adherence to schedules. People in polychronic cultures are almost never alone, even in the home, and are continually interacting with several people at once.

Nowhere is the conflict of different time patterns more evident than in the bureaucratic system of the hospital. The timing of activities within a complex system such as a large hospital is indeed an intricate task. Diagnostic centers plan their schedules; food service sets its hours; nursing plans its workload to coincide with the periods of shift rotations; and superimposed on these patterns are the demands placed on nursing staff and patients by surgery and the unscheduled rounds of medical staff. These time demands are woven into a program for each patient. The extent to which the patient's own time preferences are taken into consideration is questionable.

The story of a nineteen-year-old East Indian youth who had an extremely severe case of arthritis and was being treated in a large metropolitan rehabilitation institution illustrates the dilemma. He was considered "uncooperative" by the staff, and his participation in the rehabilitative services was minimal. One example of his "lack of cooperation," as related by the head nurse, was that he frequently refused to eat supper when it was served and drank only the tea on his tray, but later he ordered pizzas or similar foods to be brought in from restaurants. The next morning he would complain of gastrointestinal disturbances and, consequently, not be able to go to physical therapy that morning. When I talked with the patient regarding his preferences for a daily routine, he said that he did not like physical activity of any sort but recognized the need for it in his particular condition. He preferred to read in the morning and perhaps, if necessary, to engage in physical activity later in the day. In accordance with his cultural and family background, he was accustomed to tea at 5:00 p.m. (hospital suppertime) and dinner around 8:00 (the time he would have meals brought in from the outside). He was also accustomed to highly seasoned food (like pizza) and did not like the relatively bland hospital fare. Viewing this patient's activities from an outsider's perspective, I began to see that he was striving to maintain his life-style and his own activity pattern, but in so doing he was having to endure the hostility of the staff in relation to their thwarted plans for his care and he ultimately lost the benefit of the rehabilitation services for which he was hospitalized.

Time is also a symbol of status. How much discretion people have in determining the way they spend their time is an indication of their status and power. When patients are made to wait for health care services, the message is clear as to who is important and who is not. While interviewing quadriplegics regarding their evaluation of motorized wheelchairs, I met a man who found it impossible to coordinate his time pattern with that of the staff. He had become quadriplegic as a result of a fall and had been given a motorized wheelchair in an effort to mobilize him. Initially he was enthusiastic about the chair but later he hardly ever got out of bed. The nurse viewed him as a complainer, with many physical complaints. The patient's view was that he wanted to use the chair, but he was afraid to stay up for more than 3 to 4 hours because of the danger of pressure sores and he had difficulty getting assistance from the staff at the time he wanted to get up (and down). According to him, the staff preferred to get all the patients up early in the morning and then back to bed either early in the afternoon before the shift change or late in the afternoon when the next shift's staff could handle it. Neither of these times was congruent with his needs: He was not ready to get up until around 1:00 (too late, according to the morning shift workers) and was afraid that even if they got him up at that time, he might be left up too long before the evening shift workers were ready to help him back to bed. He felt that his time preferences did not fit in with the way they wanted to do their work. He acknowledged that he did have complaints of stomach pain frequently and that the pain was worse when he became upset over his situation. This patient' s mobilization was blocked by his inability to articulate his time pattern with the quantitative, task-oriented pattern of the staff. The increasing frustration he experienced was accompanied by an increase in his stomach pain and, subsequently, an increased need to stay in bed. He was caught in a vicious cycle.

There is considerable evidence that people's temporal patterns are highly individualistic and have a bearing on their response to other people, their receptivity to therapy, their ability to learn new tasks, and, consequently, their feelings about themselves. These examples represent the power struggles patients and staff get caught in when the patients are attempting to be themselves and the result impinges upon the staff's need to perform their work in a routine way. The additional time pressure placed on staff by today's emphasis on decreased length of hospitalization may place the patient's temporal pattern in further jeopardy.

SPACE-TIME BINDING

Condon (1980), after years of research on the interactional synchrony of mothers and neonates and of speakers and listeners, makes a strong case for individuals as *participants* in a complicated organization, a kind of web, of space-time: "The individuals do not create that order but participate in it. They 'live into' the forms and experiences which surround them and these forms become part of their very being" (p. 56). This description is consistent with the idea that matter is a precipitate of the underlying pattern, the implicate order.

Interactional synchrony of the movement of infants in relation to adult voices has been observed as early as 20 minutes after birth and may, according to Condon, exist in utero. The newborn's ability to entrain with the mother's speech provides a mechanism that helps to explain the bonding process. It also may help to explain the difficulties some adopted parent-child dyads experience. The child is entrained to a different rhythm, that of the natural mother, and may be out of sync with the adopted mother.

Friedman (1983) has introduced an interesting view of space-time as an indicator of self-concept. His conceptualization goes beyond the usual idea of self-concept and is presented as a measure of transpersonal development:

> A key construct . . . is the *level of self-expansiveness*, which is defined as the amount of the self which is contained within the boundary demarcating self from non-self through the process of *self-conception*. . . . the position is taken that the relationship between self and non-self is inherently unlimited. . . . The self is thus seen as inextricably embedded in the universe . . . (p. 38)

Friedman builds on Deikman's view that the self is experienced in terms of the space-time of the world, in terms of all the things included in the zone of personal organization. The sense of identity is enlarged or contracted in terms of *extension beyond the here-and-now*.

Some examples of women interviewed by graduate students as a part of their study of adult health illustrate the centrality of space-time. Data were collected in general terms in relation to the interaction of these women with their environment and were later analyzed from the standpoint of movement-space-time as manifestations of consciousness:

> **Case 1:** Mrs. V. made repeated attempts to *move* away from husband and to *move* into an educational program to become more independent. She felt she had no *space* for herself and she tried to distance herself (*space*) from her husband. She felt she had no *time* for leisure (self), was overworked, and was constantly meeting other people's needs. She was submissive to demands and criticism of her husband.
>
> **Case 2:** Mrs. K. has decreased her activities (*movement*) outside of home (such as work, and church) and appears to be separating herself from others (building up *space* around herself). Her husband is away from home most of the time. There are indications that she is taking some form of sedatives or alcohol and sleeps most of the time (altering *time*).
>
> **Case 3:** Mrs. L. is viewed as a "driving personality" (*movement*) and is very active but reluctant to *move* outside her own area. She cannot tolerate her husband, or her boss, in "her *space*." She is very controlled in her use of *time*. She cannot confide in co-workers and does not communicate openly with husband or boss.
>
> **Case 4:** Mrs. C. has very little activity outside the home (*movement/space*) except for her work. She has no private *space* ("cannot go to bathroom alone") and no *time* alone. She has no social life and finds her interactions controlled by her husband and child.

These examples were all drawn from a similar population in a semirural, middle-class setting. They all reflect a diminished sense of self as reflected in contracted, almost nonexistent space-time dimension. They illustrate the relevance of the space-time dimension in the sense of self. The point of intersection of the time, space, and movement dimensions represents the pattern of consciousness, the quality and quantity of interaction. In all of these examples the interaction was characterized by submission, resentment, and distancing, was practically nonexistent in relation to persons outside the home, and could be regarded as a low level of consciousness as defined in this model.

Kunz and Peper (1982–1983) emphasize that " . . . interpersonal interaction . . . keeps us alive." They assert that energy in all the fields (physical, vital, emotional, mental, intuitive) must be incoming, outgoing, and freely flowing, and they remind us that we are a "part of a dynamic energy pattern" of the universe. In interviews with over 2000 men who had had myocardial infarctions, Ruberman and associates (1984) found that social isolation was a major factor in risk of death. In another situation, as death nears in children with leukemia, they prefer increasing space between themselves and others (Spinetta et al., 1974). These findings raise interesting questions regarding the meaning of personal space in terms of consciousness.

West's observations of mothers of developmentally disabled children revealed a different quality of interaction and a different sense of self (West, 1984b). Even though these mothers' child care responsibilities made independent movement outside the family difficult, they compensated by activities in which the *family moved together*. These mothers tended to protect the family space from intrusion by outsiders. They equated time and space and occasionally felt that time dragged when activity was decreased; however, usually their responsibilities filled their days. They acknowledged that they could not control time and found it important to live in the "now" dimension—"one day at a time."

The interrelatedness of time and space has been explored

experimentally by DeLong (1981; DeLong & Lubar, 1979). The findings of these experiments indicate that smaller-scale environments are related to increased subjective time. DeLong and Lubar report that subjects experience time as intense and densely packed. These findings are consistent with a relatively high index of consciousness (Bentov, 1978)—the subjects' ratio of subjective time to clock time is high—and have important implications for persons whose space is restricted. Since environmental space appears to mediate one's experience of time, DeLong and Lubar are suggesting that it be investigated as a possible factor in the development of hyperkinesis. What this suggests is that variation in environmental space could be utilized in situations where heavy time/no time are considered undesirable conditions.

INTEGRATION VIA MOVEMENT

Movement is a pivotal choice point in the evolution of human consciousness. Movement is the natural condition of life. When movement ceases, one fears that life has gone out of the organism. The consciousness that characterizes any form of life is expressed in its movement. It is through movement that the organism interacts with its environment and exercises control over its interactions. It is the fullest expression of consciousness in matter. Bohm (1981) sees it as the immediate experience of the implicate order: We do not know how we move, but when we wish to go somewhere, our imagination displays the activity. When we come into being in this physical world, we exist in time and space with a limited sense of self. Through movement we expand our knowledge of ourselves and others and the environment.

Kinesthetic consciousness is identical with the manifest dimensions of the world, a "world consciousness" (Mikunas, 1974, p. 11). In this sense, movement is not thought of as a succession of bodily locations. The schema of the total dance is present in each movement. This corresponds to a holographic view of the universe in which all of space-time is captured in any one place-moment. Behnke (1974) adds that " . . . every visible or audible gesture points to and makes present an invisible or silent dimension which is the context constituting the very significance of the gesture" (p. 13) The quality, rhythm, and exchange of facial movements, eye movements, body gestures, voice, and walking gait all mirror our consciousness and reflect our attitudes and thoughts, the meaning we give reality (Gottlieb, 1982; Seagel, 1983).

The pattern of movement reflects the overall organization of the thought and feeling processes of a person. Just as muscle activity is characterized by preparation-action-recovery, so an individual's overall pattern of movement reflects this inner organization and communicates the harmony of one's pattern with the environment (Hall & Cobey, 1974). The cycle of preparation-action-recovery becomes a spiral of development of our consciousness throughout the life span.

Rhythm is basic to movement:

> At the heart of each of us, whatever our imperfections, there exists a silent pulse of perfect rhythm, a complex of wave forms and resonances, which is absolutely individual and unique, and yet which connects us to everything in the universe. (Leonard, 1978, pp. xii)

Language reflects the rhythm of one's personal tempo, and this rhythm may be reflective of both the rhythm of the person and the rhythm of the culture of which the person is a part. When one cannot establish a mutually satisfying rhythm of relating, it is difficult if not impossible to communicate. When two people are relating well, the rhythm of the speaker is shared by the listener in a kind of mutual dance of empathy. The listener is not reacting or responding to the speaker but is "one with" the speaker. At the exact fraction of a second the speaker resumes talking, the listener begins his or her series of synchronized movements (Condon, 1980).

Hall (1984) reported a problem of blacks and whites in becoming synchronized with each other and attributed this difficulty to the feel or rhythm of the talk, not the words. The differences reported may be a function of the shared rhythm of the culture, rather than factors attributable to race. Blacks and whites reared in the same culture very often find that they are on the same "wavelength." Leonard (1978) reports Paul Byers' research in which he observed the verbal exchange between the chiefs of two villages in South America. The exchange *appeared* to be an angry shouting match. He reports, however, that the timing of the exchange is very precise and reveals a synchronized talk dance. This synchronization has a biological effect of making the interactants feel good about what they're doing and about each other. Moving in synchrony with someone else, as in playing a musical instrument in an orchestra, singing in a choir, or marching in a parade, brings with it a feeling of closeness and unity with a greater whole.

The rhythm of movement is an integrating experience and has been used as such in treatment of persons with learning disabilities, who tend to have a poor sense of rhythm. Gottlieb (1982, 1983) uses a trampoline to unite motor and cognitive abilities; clients are instructed to recite the alphabet or do simple numerical calculation while jumping on a trampoline. A change in the pattern of jumping is coordinated with more complex cognitive activity, and clients are able to improve their psychomotor and cognitive awareness simultaneously. Differences in pattern of movement have also been observed in relation to mental retardation (Murdoch & Kenedi, 1981).

When one's natural movement tempo is altered, as by trauma or by diseases of the neuromusculoskeletal system, one's perception of space-time also changes. My earliest research (Newman, 1972, 1976) was based on Piaget's thesis that time is a function of movement. When subjects were required to walk at rates 30% and 50% slower than their natural walking rate, their sense of subjective time was less than while walking at their natural rate. This relationship was supported by Tompkins' (1980) research, in which she simulated restricted movement by the application of knee and ankle braces. If this sense of diminished subjective time occurs in situations of natural restrictions of movement, it implies the presence of conflicting time senses, or rhythms, among people of varying movement tempos.

Hall and Cobey (1974) see all body movement "in terms of that which is directed outward and that which is directed inward, in terms of attacking and defending, or more broadly, proceeding and yielding" (p. 6). This phenomenon was very apparent when, early in the development of specialized motorized wheelchairs, men who were long-time high-level quadriplegics regained some independent mobility. Before receiving these chairs, these men had been confined to manual wheelchairs and had been dependent on others for their movement from place to place. The specially designed controls allowed them to operate the chairs by themselves and made possible a significant increase in activities and places accessible to them. The overriding response by far was the sense of control they had recaptured over their space and time and interaction with others. They could go to visit someone when they wanted to, not when an aide was available to take them. More importantly, they could terminate that visit when it was no longer desirable to stay. Few of us stop to consider the control that movement affords us, to approach and withdraw as we please.

There are many situations in which this type of restriction of freedom occurs. The most obvious are those in which persons are incapacitated by chronic disease and no longer able to pursue their previous activities. New parents are confronted suddenly with the loss of freedom entailed with their parenting responsibilities. Others, physically able but educationally or culturally deprived, find movement out of a circumscribed space-time difficult. Even though much progress has been made in readmitting the elderly to the mainstream of society, many of our senior citizens still find certain avenues no longer open to them: their work, former companions, their family. These dimensions of their life space have become restricted.

In some of these situations individuals may feel as though they have been robbed of their time; in others they may feel as though they have too much time. In either case our time is our life. The way we experience our time is the way we experience our life, and it is inextricably linked to space and movement.

My mother's incapacitation with amyotrophic lateral sclerosis made me very much aware of what restricted mobility means in terms of space and time. Not only was my mother not free to move about in space or to control her own time, but these restrictions applied also to me, the primary caregiver. The freedom to come and go as one pleases, when one pleases, is taken for granted until circumstances render that movement impossible or unwise. Restriction of movement forces one into a realm beyond space and time. The old ways of living and relating don't work anymore. One is confronted with one's own inner resources, the quality of one's relationships, and one's ability to live in the present. The developmental task is to allow the transformation of ourselves to occur as we move beyond space and time to higher consciousness.

BEYOND SPACE-TIME

Multitudes of philosophers, artists, poets, and scientists have tried to capture the meaning of time and to learn somehow to control it. Bohm (1980) proposes that the basic element of reality is "a *moment* which, like the moment of consciousness, cannot be precisely related to measurements of space and time, but rather covers a somewhat vaguely defined region which is extended in space and has duration in time" (p. 207). Each moment has an explicate order and also enfolds all others. This would mean that each moment of our lives contains all others of all time. Just as in the earlier illustration that elements separated in space are noncausally and nonlocally related, this introduces a new notion of time. Moments separated in time are also projections of a larger interconnected reality and may present themselves in varying orders of sequencing.

Our notions of causality rely on a linear, sequential view of time, our confidence in continuity, and do not encompass the basic tenets of evolution and quantum theory, that order and reason are based on a notion of randomness (Jones, 1982). Jones asserts: "but first the point (chaotic, unified, dimensionless, timeless experience) must become the interval. How? This is the fundamental act of creation, of the movement from unmanifest to manifest" (p. 97). The notion of causality depends on a particular view of space and time, motion in time through extended space. In a nondimensional totality-point, such as Jones suggests, no causal explanation can exist, since everything is everything else. Even the idea of relationship is no longer meaningful.

Bentov's conceptualization of the relationship of subjective time to objective time (clock time) has rendered the data of my studies of perceived duration (Newman, 1976, 1982) meaningful as support for expanding consciousness across the life span. According to Bentov (1978), when an individual's subjective time is greater than objective time (say the *experience* of 4 seconds in 1 second of clock time), this ratio would indicate a higher level of consciousness than for someone whose subjective time equals clock time (1 to 1). The greater subjective time is not experienced as time racing, as one might expect when we quantify it as 4 to 1. Rather it is experienced as a kind of dilatation or stretching of time, such as one experiences in a dream state. One has the experience of having a lot of time available in a short period of clock time. Athletes have reported this kind of experience, as is depicted in this account of a quarterback's feeling that he has all the time in the world to survey the field and target his pass:

> At times, I experience a kind of clarity that I've never seen described in any football story; sometimes time seems to slow way down, as if everyone were moving in slow motion. It seems as if I have all the time in the world to watch the receivers run their patterns, and yet I know the defensive line is coming at me just as fast as ever, and yet the whole thing seems like a movie or a dance in slow motion. It's beautiful. (Brodie, cited by Smith, 1975, p. 187)

The clarity that John Brodie felt illustrates the expanded consciousness associated with expanded time.

Bentov illustrates the relationship of subjective time to objective time with rotating axes in relation to subjective space and objective space:

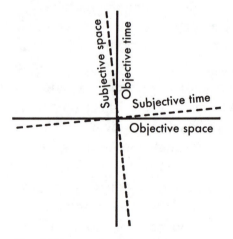

Fig. 12 Subjective Time/Objective Time

As the subjective time axis rotates toward objective space, theoretically one has all time available at all points in space *or* one's consciousness could be in all places and times at once. This conceptualization seems to me to be congruent with Bohm's moment that enfolds all others and Jones' point of unified experience.

My early experiments relating movement to perceived duration were locked into a physical, linear view of movement-space-time. However, I rather quickly became dissatisfied with time estimation as a measure of the larger concept, time, but could see it as some sort of indicator of the personal tempo, or basic rhythm, of a person. The tentative findings, that subjective time increases with age, were contrary to prevailing theory based on a physiological model. Previous work indicated that subjective time was a function of temperature/metabolic rate, both of which *decreased* with age. The data required another explanation. In terms of Bentov's index of consciousness, the data were illustrative of increasing consciousness with age (Newman, 1982). Longitudinal studies are needed to support this conclusion and are underway.

THE HIGHEST LEVEL OF CONSCIOUSNESS

Most of us can only speculate about the highest level of consciousness. Bentov (1978) suggests that "human consciousness can be taught to expand and learn how to interact with the whole spectrum of realities." There are meditative techniques that will facilitate movement into the astral realm, but Bentov warns that care must be taken not to go unprotected into this plane. An experienced teacher is required. Once emotional problems have been worked out, the evolution of human consciousness progresses to the mental level. At the mental level "the balanced mind" and the search for knowledge are dominant. The only emotion allowed is love.

Our need is to move beyond the emotional level to a high level of consciousness in which love exists. Moss (1981) equates expanded consciousness with deeper love. This kind of love:

> . . . is not something we can want . . . like we want a bicycle, or power, or even freedom from disease. This love belongs to the whole of self. . . . Those who approach naively or from an unconscious selfishness will turn back at the first experience of this love's tendency to bring forward the repressed and the lowly equally as it reveals the beautiful and the lofty. Much that we would never want to think within us will come forth in the light of these deeper forces. (p. 9)
>
> For the mature individual who is ready for this step, the art of living is the conscious loss of control, the letting go of the obsession with self, the surrender into being, the opening of the heart. (pp. 10–11)

Peck (1978) says that the experience of real love involves extending our boundaries beyond the ego:

> What transpires then in the course of many years of loving (of extending our limits) . . . is a gradual but progressive enlargement of the self, an incorporation within of the world without, and a growth, a stretching and thinning of our ego boundaries. In this way the more and longer we extend ourselves, the more we love, the more blurred becomes the distinction between the self and the world. (p. 95)

This extension of one's boundaries to incorporate and nurture another and its concomitant expansion of one's consciousness is illustrated in West's (1984b) exploration of the experience of mothers of developmentally disabled children. Expecting to find these mothers harried by their responsibility and depressed by the limitations placed on them in the care of their children, she found instead that many of these mothers considered their experience as "special" and themselves as "chosen." They considered their experience as a "growing up" period in which they learned to be more mature, more giving and understanding, and more compassionate for other people. They felt that the presence of the child was a positive influence on the whole family and gave them purpose in life.

The mothers in West's study were able to embrace their present situation and allow themselves to be transformed by it. They were able to go beyond themselves and beyond reason into a new order of reality, a new level of consciousness. At this new level defeat, failure, and vulnerability are equally as important as success, power, and gratifying relationships. Winning is not important; experiencing the moment fully is (Moss, 1981).

In our Western civilization there is a preoccupation with outer phenomena, and the reality of our inner space is largely ignored. Moss (1981) points out that "we are afraid to venture beyond a cautious high . . . and quickly reject our lows" (p. 14). Behaviors that might carry us beyond our narrow band of acceptability are banished immediately. In this way we limit the amount of energy with which we empower our consciousness and stop short of the potential to go beyond ourselves.

In this model of health it does not matter where one is in the process. There is no basis for rejecting any experience as irrelevant. The important factor is to get in touch with one's own pattern of interaction and recognize that whatever it is, the process is in progress and the experience is one of expanding consciousness.

CHAPTER 5

INTERVENTION : NONINTERVENTION

When health is conceptualized as the expansion of consciousness in a universe of undivided wholeness, intervention aimed at producing a particular result becomes a problem. To intervene with a particular solution in mind is to say we know what form the pattern of expanding consciousness will take, and we don't. Moss (1981), who declares himself a *former* general practitioner of medicine, asks where is the world going anyway, except round in circles. Somehow this bigger picture makes it easier to relax and enjoy an authentic involvement/evolvement with another person.

In order to function in the new paradigm, a model of nonintervention is needed. The old paradigm is instrumental and requires that the professional identify what is wrong and why it is wrong and then take steps to fix it. The new paradigm is relational. The professional enters into a partnership with the client with the mutual goal of participating in an authentic relationship, trusting that in the process of its evolving, both will grow and become healthier in the sense of higher levels of consciousness.

Moss (1981) asserts that the real task for us as health professionals is to stop trying to change the world in accordance with our own image of what is healthy and instead "fall toward the center of ourselves." He believes that the necessity for doing leads us into a pattern of contraction and diminished sensitivity; we must be willing to allow people to pursue their own destiny.

Vaughan (1979) agrees. She says it is impossible to know what a "successful" outcome will be other than that it is a shift from the self, from personal goals, to the universe, to a broader perspective. When this occurs, it will be manifest in congruence between inner and outer experience, harmony, inner peace, and a greater capacity for love and relatedness in the world. The health professional's awareness of being, rather than doing, is the primary mechanism of helping: ". . . being with another person, willing to participate empathically in his/her experience, without becoming identified with it and without imposing any agenda, preconceived goals, or outcomes on the process" (Vaughan, 1979, p. 28).

B. Doberneck, a nursing clinician, relates her experience in giving up her own agenda and in being with clients not to change anything but simply to be with them as they identify their concerns and the actions they want to pursue. She points out that things come up that are more central to their lives than what she might have had on her agenda. She admitted that she had to guard against a "doing" approach. It was not that she didn't do anything. In the process of her interaction with clients, she shared information regarding topics of concern to them, referred one patient to a physician on the basis of symptoms of heart disease, discussed one patient's concerns regarding the anticipated death of her spouse, and helped a grandmother deal with the developmental crisis of her young adult grandson. Doberneck observed that if she could maintain this unconditional caring relationship long enough, a shift would occur when trust had been established; the relationship then felt somehow "lighter" and the psychological and physical distancing that had been characteristic of the relationship seemed to disappear.

HOLOGRAPHIC MODEL

A holographic model of intervention appears to be consistent with the new paradigm. To comprehend this model it is helpful to review some of the basic elements of a hologram. A hologram contains an image in which the whole is written into each part; the three-dimensional image is produced by wavefront reconstruction. Light waves bouncing off an object interact with a pure light reference beam, and the resulting interference pattern is imprinted on the film. When another reference beam is projected through the film, the image of the object is recreated by the interference patterns of the film. This process is often explained by imagining the emanating waves that appear when two pebbles are thrown into water. As the waves radiate toward each other, they meet and interact and an interference pattern evolves. The interference pattern spreads and is a part of the whole of each of the previous patterns.

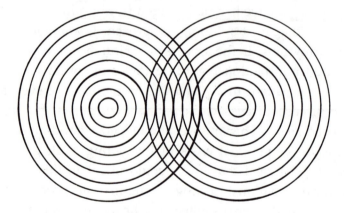

Fig. 13 Interference Pattern of Waves Emanating from two Pebbles Thrown in a Body of Water

Now substitute two people for the two pebbles and imagine *the waves radiating from each person interacting with the other pattern and becoming an interference pattern that is part of each person's pattern*:

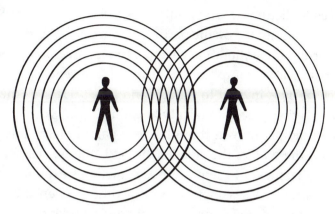

Fig. 14 Interaction Pattern of Two Persons: A Holographic Model of Intervention

The interference pattern continues and encompasses the whole environment. To be in touch with the other person and the environment, the task is to be *in touch with one's own pattern*. Jantsch (1980) cited an example from Pelletier, in which the EEG of a healer who was in the process of concentrating on a patient assumed the precise pattern of the patient's EEG. This was interpreted to mean that cognition of the patient was accomplished by *recognition out of himself*.

The observer and the observed are interpenetrating aspects of one whole. In a holographic view of the world the totality of existence is enfolded in each region of space and time. The order that has been recorded in the complex movement of electromagnetic fields (light waves) is present everywhere and enfolds the entire information of the universe in each region of space and time (Bohm, 1980).

The clearer we are in knowing ourselves, the clearer we will be in knowing other persons and the more meaningful will be our relationships. The thesis of this book is that the highest form of knowing is loving, and so we are admonished to love ourselves, a dictum not unfamiliar in spiritual teachings. Keen (1978) has commented on the partnership of science and religion in supporting the notion that each person is a microcosm of the macrocosm with the implication: "Consider the enormity of the self each of us is invited to inhabit and love." He sees the self as "the meeting place of eternity and time" (p. 88).

In a hologram, even though every part contains information about the whole, the smaller the part, the fuzzier the picture. The fuzziness of the pattern is sometimes experienced in the beginning of assessment of self or others when there is a sense of pattern or meaning that is not entirely clear. Welwood (1978), referring to Gendlin's work on focusing, compares our "felt meaning" to the interference pattern of the hologram and sees felt meaning as a manifestation of this pattern.

In the old paradigm, practice was divided into discrete parts: assessment, diagnosis, intervention. In the new paradigm there are no separate parts; the process is one of pattern recognition. There is no permanent pattern of fixed form but a continous flow of actions and movements that merge into each other. Music gives us this sense of the moving, interpenetration of many forms and relationships.

PATTERN RECOGNITION

The task in intervention is pattern recognition. This occurs, as I have suggested, by going into ourselves and getting in touch with our own pattern and through it in touch with the pattern of the person or persons with whom we are interacting. Gendlin's (1978) process of focusing is a helpful starting point. This process involves directed concentration on oneself, more specifically on the feelings one is aware of in the body. It may be a heaviness in the heart or stomach area, a pain in the shoulders or lower back, or something far more diffuse. The task is to concentrate on that feeling, to get in touch with it, and to try to explicate it by naming it. If the first name you give it does not "feel" right, you stay with it and continue to name it until your identification of the feeling coincides with the deeper nonverbal message of your body. When this congruence is reached, there is usually a total relaxing shift that occurs in your body similar to that experienced when you finally remember something that you have been blocking on. This process of focusing and relaxing releases energy for growth even when you are not conscious of what growth is occurring, and this is true when you practice the process with someone else. If you are the facilitator, you are acting like the reference beam in the hologram, making it possible for the interference pattern to emerge and for pattern recognition to occur. This process may take a while and seem to be going nowhere, but if one can be patient and trust in the unseen, evolving pattern, it will eventually emerge.

In spite of this belief that pattern recognition is more a matter of being able to "read" one's own pattern than of collecting information "external" to oneself, an assessment framework may be useful in initial efforts to identify pattern. The assessment framework developed by the nurse theorist group of the North American Nursing Diagnosis Association (NANDA) is consistent with the paradigm of health presented here. It is based on the following assumptions: (1) The pattern of a person is unitary and maintains its identity while in continuous change. (2) The human field is an energy field in constant interaction with the environmental energy field (Roy et al., 1982).

The dimensions of this assessment framework—exchanging, communicating, relating, valuing, choosing, moving, perceiving, feeling, and knowing—are considered to be manifestations of the unitary pattern. Operationalization of these terms is ambiguous and overlapping, limited by our ability to comprehend the underlying pattern. The following definitions represent my modification of those agreed upon by the theorist group:

Exchanging   interchanging matter and energy between person and environment and transforming energy from one form to another
Communicating   interchanging information from one system to another
Relating   connecting with other persons and the environment
Valuing   assigning worth
Choosing   selecting of one or more alternatives
Moving   rhythmic alternating between activity and rest
Perceiving   receiving and interpreting information
Feeling   sensing physical and intuitive awareness
Knowing   personal recognizing of self and world

These dimensions were identified by a combined approach of an inductive clustering of observations made in nursing practice and a deductive selection of crucial concepts consistent with a theoretical model of unitary human beings. The intent is that the practitioner survey the data of the client-environment interaction in terms of these dimensions in a search for the underlying pattern of these relationships (Newman, 1984).

Those who have used this framework for health assessment have found it extremely helpful in forcing one to describe a total nonjudgmental pattern of interaction at a point in space-time and thereby to abandon a dichotomous view of disease/nondisease. In its original form it provides assessment of the individual client in relation to family and community. Depending on where the focus is placed, it can provide an assessment of either the individual pattern or the family pattern or both. In addition, West (1984a) has used this framework as a basis for describing the human relationships that make up the pattern of interaction of a community.

As a number of nursing practitioners have commented, this assessment framework makes explicit what nurses have been doing intuitively all along but have not been able to explain. In my early days in nursing practice I was convinced that the process of nursing was identifiable, but when challenged to explain the assessment-intervention process hypothetically in relation to specific medical problems, I could not come up with anything very specific.

The problem was the hypothetical nature of the question. Nursing diagnosis/intervention is based on the unique configuration of each person-environment situation. It is impossible to project that pattern until you are in an actual situation interacting with the specific configuration present at that moment. Masson (1985) supports this difficulty of articulating the language of nursing, as compared with the language of the technology of medicine: "The practice of nursing cannot be lifted out of its cultural *context*, nor can it always be understood except in term of *the individual nurse-patient relationship*" (p. 72) (emphasis added).

Assessment of a person-environment situation according to the dimensions of the NANDA framework yields data relevant to the model of health as expanding consciousness. The entire perspective of the assessment framework focuses on interaction and therefore yields data that describe the quantity and quality of interaction with the environment, i.e., consciousness as defined in this model. Use of this framework facilitates the emergence of the pattern of the person-family-community in a natural, unformatted way. The data can then be viewed from the standpoint of movement-space-time patterns of consciousness.

RHYTHM

Rhythm is a basic characteristic of pattern and a powerful factor in interpersonal relations. Pelletier (1978) recognized the importance of timing in client relationships. He drew an analogy of twirling balls on the end of a string. The point at which a ball is released determines the direction it will take. Being able to wait until the client is ready to move may be difficult; allowing the client to move in his or her own direction may be even more difficult.

The rhythm of talking is an important consideration in intervention. The pauses in talking may be more relevant than the words. One encounter group technique involves persons forming two concentric circles, with the inner circle facing out and the outer circle facing in. Instructions are to face a partner and say "Hello," to which the partner responds with "Hello." This exchange is repeated several times until participants are instructed to move on to the next person in the circle, and the greetings are again exchanged. This simple experiment is very revealing in that after you have gone full circle, perhaps more than once, you have a pretty good idea of which persons in the circle you can relate to and which ones you definitely do not like relating to. I submit that one of the distinguishing factors is the rhythm of the "conversation."

The person who interrupts a meaningful pause may be squelching an important idea or may never hear an important message that was forthcoming. We often think of the beats of the music or the utterances of a voice as the structure of the rhythm, but the nature of the pauses, or the silences between, are equally germane. Watson (1976) reinforces the importance of the silence between utterances in the lesson he learned from the djuru, an Indonesian native who was able to listen underwater to locate fish and predict tidal waves. The djuru instructed

Watson to put his head underwater and listen. Watson relates
the conversation:

> "What did you hear?"
> "Nothing."
> "That was my trouble too."
> "What?"
> "I could not hear it."
> "Hear what?"
> "Nothing."

Watson continues:

> I could not teach myself to listen to the silence. The djuru can do this.
> He is trained to listen intently to nothing, because the secrets lie in the
> spaces between the sounds. He is able to listen when all is quiet and
> to look when there is nothing to see.
> I remembered . . . my insistence on being told exactly what each of the
> fish sounded like. He had made up metaphors to keep me happy, and
> they had. But now I felt rather ashamed.
> [He] watched my awareness grow, and he nodded sympathetically.
> A kingfisher swept by overhead, cutting across the lagoon with deep,
> irregular wingbeats, and it was only in the brief pause between each
> flurry of feathers and the next that I could be sure of the cool cerulean
> blue of its back.
> Long after it disappeared into the mangroves, I could still hear its loud
> rattling cry. It is a very distinctive sound which fills my head with the
> message "Kingfisher calling." But it was only in the silent moment
> between one proclamation and the next that I had time to think about
> the bird. It was only in the pauses that I was able to reflect on the
> relationship between the bird and me. (pp. 196–197)

The importance of attending to the silence between signals is
crucial to getting in tune with one's inner voice, the pattern of
oneself, one's consciousness. Watson's decription of the djuru
is a vivid portrayal of how one can become receptive to the
larger pattern:

> There is no known sense organ that can give a man [sic] underwater
> the capacity for locating things precisely in the dark, or for responding
> appropriately to the precursors of a seismic wave. I believe he [the djuru]

was able to do these things because he turned his whole body on and tuned in completely to the entire spectrum of information. He listened to the waves and heard not only their news but signals in the silence between them. He measured the intervals and established a beat produced by interference between these waves and others elsewhere. And in this way he put his consciousness in a position to transcend the physical limits of information transfer. (p. 199)

PERSONAL TRANSFORMATION

The health professional who seeks to practice in this new paradigm faces personal transformation. The current health care organization is dominated by the old paradigm, one that views health as the absence of disease and dictates particular actions en masse in an effort to overcome disease. The health professional committed to a paradigm of a pattern of expanding consciousness will repeatedly recognize that the "old rules" are not working and be compelled to seek new patterns of practice. The pathway is uncertain and the feeling is unsure. Those who have gone before us assure us that in letting go and experiencing the moment fully the transformation will take place, and through us others will find a new level of integration and growth.

CHAPTER 6

FROM OLD PARADIGM TO NEW

Why is it that people can rarely identify their nurse? If asked, they can usually tell you who their doctor is, or their dentist, or their attorney, or their hairdresser, but what about their nurse? In spite of the many stories that are told of a particular nurse having served some crucial role in another person's life, the nurse somehow remains an anonymous, short-term player. Nurses seem to function in dispensable, exchangeable slots. Nurses as a group are important, but nurses as individuals have little identity.

Individual nurses do have specific contributions to make to individual patients. There have been many times that I, as a person in need of health care, wondered to myself, *outloud,* "Where is my nurse?!" I know where to turn because I have friends who are nurses. But what about people who don't? Where is their nurse? Only in the hospital? Nurses are beginning to offer their services in consultation directly to patients, but at this writing there are still very few listed in the Yellow Pages except in the form of businesses geared to provide traditional medical home care to the ill or disabled. I am encouraged that more and more nurses are offering their services directly to the public in ways consistent with the new paradigm of health. Direct reimbursement of nursing services from the usual sources of health care financing, however, is not commonly available; therefore, access to individual nurses' services is limited. Some background regarding nursing's position within the health care arena may be helpful.

THE NURSING PROFESSION: CENTER OF CONFLICT

Ever since the nursing profession opted to function primarily within the hospital structure, it has been caught in the bind of serving three masters: the organizational needs of hospital administration, the medical care directives of physicians, and the individual patient care needs as determined by the nurse's own professional judgment. These expectations/demands are not always congruent. The responsibility of hospital administration is to run a business, and the priority is to do so with efficiency and cost effectiveness; nurses are employees of the hospital and, therefore, share this responsibility. The responsibility of physicians is the medical diagnosis and treatment of the patients they have admitted; their priority is the implementation of the prescribed regimen for their patients. Nurses have a responsibility to perform certain delegated medical tasks. Each patient enters the system with his or her own pattern of relationships in conjunction with the reason for hospitalization. The nurse's primary responsibility is to recognize the total pattern of the patient's response to the particular situation at hand and to act accordingly. The position of the nurse is one of trying to balance all three sets of expectations; the result may be visualized as three forces pulling on the nurse in different directions:

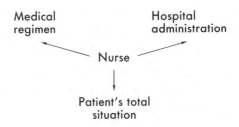

Fig. 15 Nurse as Center of Conflicting Demands

There is no wonder that hospital nurses experience so much conflict and burnout. Bound in space-time, but with no space or time to call their own, staff nurses have no real individual identity or authority. What power the nurse has attained has been accomplished by co-opting the power of hospital administration or the physician. The paradigm of practice has been one of efficiency in carrying out the dictates of the medical model. There has been little room in the system for the paradigm of health set forth in this book. The conflict and distress that many nurses have experienced in practice stem from the contradictions inherent in the two paradigms. The power of the medical model is such that, in a pinch, it predominates, and the nurse feels diminished in terms of her or his nursing responsibility to the patient.

A TEAM APPROACH

From time to time I have wondered why team nursing, a concept introduced in the early sixties, didn't work—at least not on a large scale. It seemed to me to have the potential for combining the different talents of various levels of nursing personnel in creative ways for the benefit of patients and the satisfaction of staff. The idea was to establish a highly qualified nurse as responsible for the nursing care of a certain number of patients with the assistance of a team of other nurses, associate nurses, and auxiliary personnel. The team leader's administrative responsibility was focused on patient care, not on unit management, as had been the case of head nurses. The crucial task of the team leader was to determine the best match of the nursing needs of the patients with the qualifications of the staff. The goal was to have the entire team work together in a coordinated way for the benefit of each patient assigned to their team.

An experience I had as a senior student during that time may help to illustrate this point. I was introduced to the concept of team nursing as part of a practicum and was given the opportunity to implement it. The first day my co-team leader and I made assignments the only way we knew: so many patients of such-and-such a level of severity of illness to so many nurses, with certain functional assignments directed to the associate nurses and aides—a quantitative approach. At the end of the day we had accomplished our tasks but with little sense of satisfaction of having really related to the staff or the patients on the unit in a meaningful way. The "old rules" were not working. We decided to throw out our fairly set ideas of how work should be distributed and began to really evaluate one by one what each patient (as a whole person) needed and which staff member(s) had the education and ability to relate to those needs—a qualitative approach. We ended up with a completely different kind of distribution. The most highly qualified staff nurse and one aide were assigned totally to one long-term patient who had been receiving "routine" physical care by the least-prepared staff members. The patient was immobilized on a Stryker frame, had large pressure sores, and was not a particularly attractive person to whom to relate. Having used a large proportion of our team for this one patient, we then had to assign much larger numbers of less "needy" patients to the remaining staff. We struggled with making this assignment, fearing that the highly qualified nurse might initially resent the tasks involved and that the other staff members might see her load as "light" compared to theirs if only numbers were considered.

But at the end of the day it had worked! The nurse assigned to this patient committed herself to relate to the patient on a person-to-person human level while at the same time addressing his physical needs, with the help of the aide. She began to identify his higher-level needs for interaction with his environment and arranged for changes in his situation that facilitated more interaction. Her task was exhausting, but at the end of the day she and everybody else on the team knew that her efforts had made a difference. Because we were a team, we all shared in both her difficulties and her success.

That experience convinced me that the integrative approach of team care was a meaningful, holistic way to deal with the complexities of patient care. It utilized the abilities of each staff member to best advantage, providing job satisfaction for them, and provided individualized care to patients. The key to its implementation, or lack thereof, was the degree to which the concept was understood and incorporated by the team leader. I don't believe this understanding was prevalent enough among educators and practitioners during that period to make a noticeable impact. Admittedly, as Manthey (1980) has pointed out, there were still other problems to be solved, such as discontinuity of care as one team leader was exchanged for another and the cumbersome process of communication within and between teams. In addition, the nursing team was functioning parallel and subordinate to the medical staff. The authority of the nurse responsible for the patient's care could always be overridden by medical authority. Eventually the concept was lost and the organization of teams reverted to the previous functional, quantitative approach rather than a holistic, qualitative approach. The only way out of that form of fragmentation and alienation, some people thought, was a "back to basics" move.

BACK TO BASICS

In the early seventies nursing leaders began to emphasize the concept of primary care, meaning that one nurse has the primary responsibility for the planning and implementation of the nursing care for a particular patient for the entire period of hospitalization. In some instances, this concept was construed to mean that the primary nurse "did everything" for the patient, without the assistance of auxiliary personnel. What it does mean is that the primary nurse has 24-hour responsibility for the patient's care, participates in the care as necessary to gain a full understanding of the patient's situation, and determines what nursing care the patient is to receive. When the primary nurse is not assuming the direct care, other nurses and auxiliary personnel follow the primary nurse's directions for care (Manthey, 1980). In spite of widespread support for the one-to-one concept of primary care, this approach has not been fully implemented and therefore has not fulfilled its promise.

CYCLES OF CHANGE

Understanding of the changes that have taken place thus far in the organization of nursing service is facilitated by Ainsworth-Land's theory of the cycles of growth (Ainsworth-Land, 1982; Land, 1973). The first stage of the cycle of growth is characterized by formative activity. The phenomenon is in the process of becoming itself and establishing its identity. In nursing, as in medicine, early practitioners functioned primarily as solo practitioners in the home, a situation in which there was a person-to-person relationship for the purpose of nurturing the health of the patient and one in which individual practitioners were in control of and responsible for their practice. The change that takes place is accretive, i.e., it expands itself and becomes more of itself.

The second stage of development is characterized as normative, a stage in which the system in interaction with the environment loses some of the authority and expansion of the first stage and develops a competitive, persuasive stance in trying to establish and maintain its own territory. Nurses, in response to rapid developments in medical technology and emphasis on hospital care, moved into the hospital setting, becoming employees of the hospital, rather than the patient, and subordinates of medicine. Hospital nursing became separated from home care nursing. Nurses then began a long period of filling in the gap of medical technology, serving the needs of the bureaucratic institution and at the same time trying to fulfill nursing's original role of one-to-one "laying on of hands" in the care of ill patients. The demand for this type of care increased, and in order to get all of the tasks completed, they were doled out as tasks per se: medicines to be distributed, blood pressures to be taken, and so on. A large majority of nurses began to lose the essence of nursing, the one-to-one personalized care of earlier days.

In the third stage, the integrative stage, the system begins to relate to other systems in the environment in a cooperative, mutual way. A partnership approach becomes the predominant way of life. Sometimes in this stage change takes place very rapidly; persons involved fear the loss of their previous secure status, and they seek to move "back to basics," rather than onward in the evolutionary cycle of transformation (Ainsworth-Land, 1982).

There was a rather short-lived effort to go beyond the functional delivery of care to a more integrated team approach of combining individual, personalized care with some functional assignments: the concept of team nursing introduced in the early sixties. However, medicine was not a partner to this approach, and the concept never really became a reality. Stage 2 participants are very reluctant to relinquish the territory they have gained in order to establish a cooperative approach. Neither educators nor practitioners in the early sixties were able to let go of the Stage 2 type of hierarchy of organization in which one person, usually the most highly educated, was in charge and delegated tasks of medical technology to other members of the staff in an assembly-line fashion. It was difficult to shift from this approach to incorporate the idea that patients had to be viewed as wholes and that the staff, in order not to be segmented and alienated by their work, had to be fully cognizant of how their responsibilities contributed to the whole of the care for the patients.

Primary nursing was a "back to basics" attempt to reestablish personal responsibility on the part of the nurse in direct relationship to the client. It has not addressed fully, however, the basic problem of lack of ongoing professional responsibility and authority of the nurse for a patient's care. The primary nurse is still bound in space-time to the particular period of hospitalization in question, to the particular institution of employment, and to fulfilling at least partially the routine responsibilities of delegated medical care. If nursing is to fulfill its responsibility to the patient in implementing a paradigm of practice that recognizes disease as a manifestation of evolution toward higher consciousness, it will have to move forward to a system that integrates the valuable contributions of previous approaches and frees the nurse to function as a full partner in health care. The conflict being experienced by nurses in relation to their responsibility to patients, hospital administration, and medicine may be just the empowering fluctuation that could transform these forces into the integrative stage.

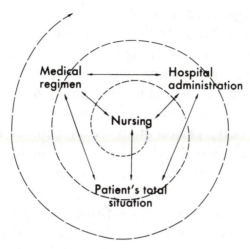

Fig. 16 Nursing as Integrative Force

NURSING IN THE NEW PARADIGM

Capra (1982) points out that nurses are perhaps the best prepared to offer health care within the new paradigm of health—health based on pattern recognition and facilitation rather than on diagnosis and treatment of disease. Nurses should be at the forefront, or perhaps *interface*, of health care offerings. In order to do this, there must be recognition and endorsement that nurses are responsible providers of essential health care services. Such recognition would be manifest in direct economic remuneration for activities falling within the realm of the new paradigm.

Currently nurses are functioning in both the old and the new paradigms, and two different roles for nurses are needed. The old paradigm is based on the concept of health as the absence of disease. This is predominantly the medical model. Activity is directed toward identifying the disease and its cause and eliminating the disease via surgical or medical means. The disease is regarded as an entity in and of itself and as the enemy to be defeated. Nurses in this model function as technicians for the purpose of implementing the medical regimen, observing and communicating the patient's condition, and providing assistance to the patient and family with activities of daily living.

The new paradigm is based on health as the undivided wholeness of the person in interaction with the environment. Nursing practice is directed toward recognizing the *pattern* of that interaction and accepting it as a process of evolving consciousness. Disease is regarded as a manifestation of that pattern, not an entity external to it. Disease can be seen as an overt manifestation (the explicate order) of the underlying unseen pattern (the implicate order). Understanding of this underlying pattern will facilitate change to higher levels of consciousness. Nurses functioning in this model have as their objective an authentic involvement of themselves with the patient in a mutual relationship of pattern recognition and augmentation. Impetus for this kind of involvement includes situations of childbirth and parenting, caring for a loved one with long-term illness, or trying to cope with one's own health concerns.

In a situation in which the old paradigm prevails, the nurse occupies a central, pivotal position between the patient and the larger health care system. It is a short-term responsibility involving performance of tasks related to the immediate medical regimen and self-care. At the same time, it involves being fully present with the patient in the immediate moment, sensing into the patient's field and facilitating the insight of pattern recognition. Nurses have been doing this without knowing exactly what they were doing or how to describe it. Patients have experienced it without knowing exactly what they were experiencing. The nurse and the patient, as participants in a greater whole, are not "nurse" and "patient." They are not separate persons. They are persons experiencing the pattern of consciousness formed by their interaction. Their relationship is based not only on problems and solutions (old paradigm) but is a manifestation of the evolving consciousness of the whole (new paradigm). An integrated team approach is needed, with the physician as a member of the team, not outside and above it as has been the usual case.

Another role is needed in order for nurses to function fully in the new paradigm. Currently nurses function in segments of space-time, either in the hospital during the acute phase of illness, in the home or extended facility for rehabilitative or long-term care, or in other agencies organized for specific time-bound purposes. Nurses need to be free to relate to patients in an ongoing partnership that is not limited to a particular place or time. Patients should be able to choose their nurse in the same way they choose their physician or dentist (perhaps they would choose them as a health professional team) and embark on the task of recognizing and facilitating their own changing patterns of health.

Education for this "primary" nurse would revolve around the concept of pattern: pattern as substance, pattern as process, and pattern as method. The learning process itself would be one of pattern recognition—extracting meaningful patterns from the confusion of large amounts of information input (Hart, 1978). Human development from the standpoint of a unitary view of human beings in a holographic model of the universe would be an underlying theme. Health would encompass the prevailing and emerging concepts of health. A major consideration would be the task of integrating the various approaches to health care within an integrated model of mutuality. Personal development of the student/practitioner would be paramount.

Ainsworth-Land (1984) points out that in third phase development everything changes: "Those things that lay outside of the limits, things that were previously out of bounds, begin to be integrated into the system. The untried and unfamiliar, rather than being rejected, now become the most important resource for continuing development." I see nursing as being that important resource for the continuing development of health care as we move into the integrative third phase. Being at the center of the intersection of the forces of the health care industry, nursing is in position to bring about the fluctuation within the system that will shift the system to a new, higher order of functioning. All evolutionary processes involve conflict between two opposing forces; a third force, in this case nursing, can bring about reconciliation of the conflict.

CHAPTER 7

KNOWLEDGE DEVELOPMENT
IN THE NEW PARADIGM

A paradigm of pattern requires a method of inquiry that will reveal pattern. The search for new alternatives in the methodology of knowledge development is apparent in nearly every field of social science. The nursing literature is replete with calls for a holistic, dynamic approach to knowledge development, an approach consistent with the basic philosophical assumptions and practice realities of the discipline.

The apparent clash between an analytical, inferential approach and an immediate, direct understanding of the pattern of a person is not new. Allport (1961) recognized the dilemma in the early sixties and was adamant that the scientific approach is necessary but incomplete without perception of the individuality of patterning:

> Inference theorists tell us that the conditions for knowing any "particular" are fulfilled only when its "universal" or class membership is recognized. This . . . means in effect that we cannot know Peter or Paul unless we fit him into stock-sized clothes. It means that we can know Peter only insofar as we can code him. He is, let us say, a white Protestant, a college male, mesomorphic in build, who has a hundred scores on a hundred personality tests, and can be tagged with general conceptual labels, such as *cordial, ardent, intense, extroverted.* All these classes, so the inference theories tell us, constitute Peter. But do they? The unit that is Peter has disintegrated into a mere powder of concepts. The continuity of Peter has been broken into discontinuous and static categories. His life . . is reduced to my conceptual furniture . . There is no way of reconstructing the true mobility and pattern of Peter from this debris of concepts. (pp. 531–532)

The role of inference is especially apparent when there is a hitch in the course of comprehension. When Peter puzzles me by his behavior, I am likely to ask, "Now what made him do that?" It was an act incompatible with my previous perception of pattern. I desire to repair the structure. I seek parallel conduct from the stores of my previous experience. But even while I try one analogy after another, and draw tentatively this inference and that, my interest is always channeled toward a patterned understanding of Peter as a single individual. (p. 546)

The solution to the dilemma, according to Allport, is to find a conciliatory approach by which we establish a method that provides both knowledge *about* people and an understanding *of* them. Search for such a method is of paramount importance as we move into the new paradigm.

Vaill (1984–1985), in criticizing the traditional models of management, asserts that "the American behavioral sciences don't amount to much as guides to action" (p. 40), that little if anything is done as a consequence of "knowledge." The problem with the old method of science, according to Vaill, is a "facts and methods" approach:

The facts and methods of modern behavioral science don't deal with the things that matter to more and more people in action roles today. Ethics matter. Feelings matter. Community matters. The human spirit matters. (p. 41)

The crux of action is meaning, and it precludes a paradigm of reason that detaches the observer from the observed. In situations where quick decisions and action are required, the person involved finds himself/herself in a situation of not knowing exactly what one wants to achieve or what means there are to achieve it. Action involves extemporization and is not for those who enjoy the mechanistic, hypotheticodeductive logic of the old paradigm. The old paradigm is about the general case. The new paradigm of action and being is about specific persons in specific situations.

These concerns are particularly relevant to nursing situations: the assessment of specific persons and action within specific, unpredictable situations. Vaill (1984–1985) suggests what he calls "process wisdom," or "being in the world with responsibility," as an alternative to the knowledge gained from the old paradigm. The themes of process wisdom involve openness and relationality:

> [W]e are talking about personal expressiveness; about a dynamic, holistic phenomenon not easily or fruitfully broken into elements and lists of key factors; that the process of understanding such a phenomenon and the process of improving the effectiveness of those who practice it cannot be a matter of objectivist science. (p. 46)

It involves the capacity to be fully conscious of one's involvement with other consciousnesses. It also involves something beyond what is known materially, a knowledge that what one is doing is somehow right.

Bohm (1980) repeatedly emphasizes the inseparability of the process of thought and the content of thought. There are certain fundamental changes in the way we think about things brought about by quantum theory:

> A centrally relevant change in descriptive order required in quantum theory is thus the dropping of the notion of analysis of the world into relatively autonomous parts, separately existent but in interaction. Rather, the primary emphasis is now on *undivided wholeness*, in which the observing instrument is not separable from what is observed. (p. 134)

We previously thought that new orders of thinking occur only occasionally, as in revolutionary periods, when old processes break down, but perception of new orders, according to Bohm, can take place anytime. We need to be continually ready to drop old notions: "understanding the fact by assimilating it into new orders can become . . . the normal way of scientific research" (p. 141).

Whyte (1974) points out that physical theory has advanced by seeking unified laws covering apparently diverse phenomena. This point is particularly relevant to the model of health being proposed: the unity of the apparently diverse phenomena of disease and nondisease. Previously the scientific rule has been to search for invariants. Now the task is to identify processes in which single less-ordered systems are unified into one well-ordered unit. This view focuses on relationships rather than substances—changing *patterns of relations*.

Davis (1982) remarks that "we are studying a complex, multifaceted, and often changing phenomenon which is not to be comprehended by old-fashioned atomistic approaches" (pp. 16–17). She agrees with Condon (1980) that participants act in synchrony and cannot be viewed in an action-reaction mode. They are coacting, moving in shared rhythms, and therefore we must learn to look at the interaction rhythm, something that cannot be seen when observing one person at a time.

The era of the scientific method can be regarded as a necessary stage of nursing's growth as a practice discipline. It has taught us to beware of our biases. Yet now we can let go of the false dichotomy of investigator-subject, recognize the impossibility of controlling the environment, and engage in participatory investigations in which subjects (clients) are our partners, our coresearchers, in our search for health patterns.

Heron (1981) refers to this view as the paradigm of cooperative inquiry. If we value self-determination and active participation in practice, then that value applies equally to research. The most authentic encounter one has with another person is when that person is encountering oneself. Heron stresses the primacy of interpenetrating attention for the development of valid social knowledge. In an interactive, dialectical process, there can be no subject-object split: The concept of "objective" is obsolete, but so also is the concept of "subjective." Validity is a function of the relationship of the knower and the known; it is "we" knowledge.

Heron makes a case for presentational construing, asserting that it includes and transcends propositional construing. Presentational construing includes form, color, and size; it portrays a sequence of presentations as a total process, as in listening to music or seeing the flight of a bird. It is a spatiotemporal whole that transcends the immediate space and time and is reminiscent of Bohm's description of the implicate order. Heron does not dismiss a propositional approach as irrelevant:

> Too much propositional construing blinds researchers to the gestures of being. Too much presentational construing keeps the archives of propositional knowledge empty . . . (p. 31) . . . true propositions are asserted by those who know how properly to symbolize in words shared experiences of shared value . . . (p. 32)

The latter point alludes to one aspect of the method endorsed by Heron that interpretations of experience should be checked out with the subject as coresearcher, one who is functioning fully as an intelligent human being. In a pattern model, we are reminded that the pattern is subject to change and that the interpretation is rarely if ever completed. All phenomena in the model are equally important; the relationships between the phenomena are crucial.

This move from normative to integrative functioning is uncertain and frightening (Ainsworth-Land, 1982). I have moved from early controlled experimental investigations in a laboratory setting through various stages of quasiexperimental and descriptive design to my most recent endeavor, a community investigation involving the subjects/participants as coinvestigators. As I experience the anxiety/uncertainty of the beginning phase of this investigation, I at times long for the safety of a neat, controlled experimental design.

But there is no turning back. We, along with the entire

spectrum of health professions, are already in the process of the integrative stage of growth. Perhaps not everyone will want to come along, at least not right away. Those of us on the frontier (or maybe some would call it the fringe) may find that we have more in common with those out front in other disciplines than we do within our own discipline. That is characteristic of an integrated approach. In the process it is important, however, to maintain our sense of identity and history in order that we may incorporate the knowledge and experience of the previous stages in the next level of development.

The old paradigm embraces a hierarchical structure. The new paradigm specifies flexible relationships and necessitates the breaking up of old connections to make room for mutuality. The current upheavals in the organization of health services and in our views about science provide fertile ground for the development of new patterns of relationships.

CHAPTER 8

BECOMING PARTNERS

Becoming partners with other health professionals means becoming partners ourselves. Possibly because the nursing profession is composed primarily of women, who have been socialized differently from men, we have not learned to function very well as a team.

However, this is changing. In a recent speech to nursing administrators, Manthey (1985) addressed the issue of self-respect and of not allowing others within the work setting to derogate fellow nurses. She exhorted nurses to "stand up" for each other:

> It is incumbent on us to understand that it is not OK under any circumstances for a physician to yell at a nurse. I often hear a young staff nurse say, "Well, I don't mind when he [sic] yells at me when I'm doing something wrong, but when he yells at me when I haven't done anything wrong, that's when I want to cry." Who says anyone can yell at anyone even when they have done something "wrong"? It is up to us to decide how long this is going to continue. If the physician is yelling at a nurse, then the nurse has decided to accept it. It is time for us to say we are not going to accept it anymore. We don't need to experience abuse. It is no longer appropriate for a staff nurse to accept abusive behavior from a physician. Not even when she has made a mistake. Yelling, by dictionary definition, is abusive behavior. When it occurs, excuse yourself and leave. Nurses tend to become immobilized when a physician starts yelling. They can't seem to walk away. One of the hospitals in California developed an alternative to walking away. They call it Code 66. When a physician starts yelling at a nurse and the nurse is unable to walk away, someone nearby pages Code 66 over the loud speaker—"Code 66–Unit 5C"—and all the available nurses in the hospital come to 5C in support of the nurse. It is not OK for staff nurses to accept

abuse; it is not OK for staff nurses to be in tears; it is not OK and we've got to change it.

Manthey's point was that in order for nurses to participate as full members of the health care team and make risk-taking decisions appropriate to the situation, there must be support from within nursing.

A relatively new organization has arisen in nursing called Cassandra: Radical Feminist Nurses Network. Its purpose is to nurture support, encouragement, and connection for women who are creating a woman-centered reality in nursing. The name is explained as follows:

> The name CASSANDRA is a tribute to Florence Nightingale who wrote an essay titled *Cassandra* in 1852. She states: "Why have women passion, intellect, moral activity—these three—and a place in society where no one of the three can be exercised?" Like the mythical Cassandra, Nightingale possessed the gift of prophesy and despaired at not being heard. We are dedicated to re-creating the Cassandra myth by providing a place where the passion, intellect and moral activity of women who are nurses can be voiced and heard.
>
> The word "radical" is defined as going to the root or origin. The word "feminist" reflects a woman-centered world view. We use these terms to convey our commitment to theory and action grounded in the reality of women's experience in nursing and in health care. A "network" is a unified structure formed of the visible and invisible. (Cassandra, 1983)

Other networking is occurring. Kane (1985) tells of a support group that originated out of her need for "nursing":

> About five years ago. . ., I was very sick and called my friend Susan for some loving care. She came and "nursed" me dearly and soon we were joined by Helen and Kathy. Since I was really down they called my long-time friend, Susan-Marie . . . and we all talked to her. Though physically it took me a few weeks to recover, all that good energy helped me that night and on through the healing process. . . . the night I was sick, the feeling was expressed that we deserved to be able to rely on this type of nurturing in our lives.

Later the group committed themselves to stay connected with each other "over the long haul." Even though they all live in different parts of the country now, they have a commitment to meet once a year and to maintain ongoing support through letters and phone calls.

I have experienced a similar need in my role as an educator-scientist. Most of my career I have worked alone and *felt* alone in my pursuit of scholarly endeavors. But recently I realized that I was tired of working alone. I was envious of people I saw on television who had teamed up for various endeavors and seemed to be enjoying their work together so much. The sense of comaraderie and of being involved in something bigger than themselves was exciting. This feeling of teamwork came across in the television series "M.A.S.H." and appeared to be true of its cast and camera crews in the production of the show. The message is that it is possible to feel a connectedness and mutual sharing in your work. I wanted to experience that.

I approached another faculty member about the possibility of our teaming up. She was mildly interested but hesitant, and I felt I could sense her fear that our collaboration would detract from her own interests and goals. Then one busy day over a cup of coffee, I shared some of my concerns/needs with two other colleagues. There was a rush of excitement and involvement as we shared our desire to be part of something bigger than ourselves. They too were tired of the drudgery of hammering out their personal professional responsibilities alone. They felt they *had* to do the things they were doing—research, writing, etc.—to survive in academia, but there was not much joy in it.

The more we considered the prospect of joining forces, the more excited we felt. We agreed to set aside a time to get together (even in the midst of our newfound fun, one of us questioned whether or not we could afford the time!) and invited the first person I had contacted to join us.

We met with the idea in mind that maybe we could combine our varied backgrounds, interests, and abilities into a research project. (What else is there?!) But before long we realized the underlying reason the four of us had gotten together was not because of similar research interests—they were, in fact, rather different—but because we each felt a sense of respect, trust, and affection for the others. We just liked each other, and that seemed like a good basis for forming a team.

We spent quite a bit of time during our first sessions together sharing our values about what we wanted out of our alliance and what fears we had about it. At one point I became very annoyed with one of our group because she seemed to be diverting the discussion from values we had shared and agreed upon and was, from my point of view, obstructing the process. We talked about my feelings/her feelings and accepted the fact that each of us was there purposely, that is, we all agreed in the beginning that even though we were so diverse, we were a good fit. What we needed to do was understand what was happening. Then the other person had a sudden insight regarding her behavior and realized that what she was doing was something she did in larger groups as well, not intentionally but as a defensive move. Each of us had similar revelations about ourselves as we shed our usual defensive ways of behaving in group and leveled with each other. The excitement of becoming more authentically ourselves and more direct in our communications grew.

Although at many meetings we discussed some semi-planned topic that was relevant to us at the time, the agenda increasingly became no-agenda. We began to trust that whatever each of us brought to the group was right for the moment.

The enthusiasm and growth that each of us felt spilled over into our other faculty and student relationships. Students in particular picked up on the meaningfulness of this process as a means of faculty support. We named ourselves Tetra for the four of us. We began to visualize a network of tetra upon tetra— each of us forming other tetra groups and they in turn forming still more.

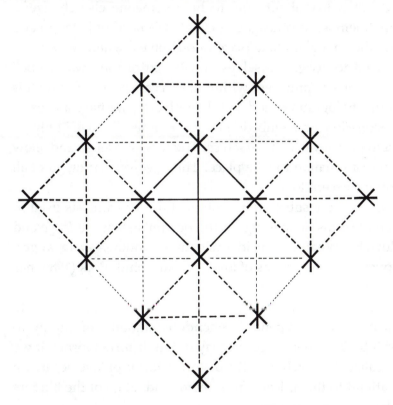

Fig. 17 Tetra Upon Tetra

As I mention our Tetra group to other groups of nurses, the concept has considerable meaning and appeal. We are not out to change anything in any particular way except for us to be more authentic in everything we do and to experience meaning and connectedness while we do it. Then, if that catches on . . .

LETTING GO

With most things it's hard to know where to begin. Not so with transformation. Transformation begins with oneself. We need not worry about how to help someone else change: a family member, a colleague, a client. We need only let go and allow the change to take place in ourselves, wherever we are. We need to accept ourselves and let go of the "way to be" admonitions so prevalent within health care circles. Seeing this within a holographic model of the universe, we have all space-time-consciousness embedded in each of us. We need only attend to the universe of ourselves. The task is to let go and allow the transformation to take place. This involves letting go of all emotions except love.

Love is the substrate for all emotion. It manifests itself in different forms depending on the person's ability to *let go* and let love be. What we consider negative emotions—hate, anger, jealousy—are distortions of love: love in a bind. Peck (1983) has defined evil as the opposite or negative end of the spectrum of love. The love is there. The person just does not know how to let it out and so expends tremendous amounts of energy to hold it back. It then forces its way out in distorted forms. If we can realize this, each time the distorted forms of love occur, we can attend to them, learn from them, and let go of the binders we have placed on love.

The understanding of sound, according to Swami Chetanananda (1985), is a means of liberation from the control of emotions such as anger:

Instead of articulating that vibration (the vibration that manifests itself as anger), or even *thinking the thought that the vibration evokes*, one simply *feels* the vibration fully. Two things then happen: (a) one attains a detachment from the emotional reaction the vibration evokes, and (b) the power behind that vibration forces one to a higher level of consciousness. Since the vibration is only a strong energy, if it is not reacted to but simply absorbed as an energy, it will promote the individual to a new level of awareness.

In order to do this it is necessary to let go of all judgment. As soon as we judge ourselves or others, we bind off the emotion, categorize it, so that it is unavailable to us to learn from.

Take, for instance, conflict. Many of us avoid conflict at any cost. We push it away, hide it, refuse to acknowledge it. We are afraid it will destroy us. In a sense, it will. If we admit it, it will reveal the true nature of what is going on and allow us to incorporate it and move beyond it—be transformed by it—and so the old me *is* destroyed. The process of acknowledging conflict, instead of binding energy, releases it for transformation.

Moss (1981) calls for an unconditional love, an embracing of all experience, a valueless state of awareness. Such a state replaces varying intensities of mood and uncontrolled emotion and lifts the energy to a finer, more radiant quality. He cautions:

> We would rather believe that love is something we can do, than something that destroys our doing and takes us into another dimension. Transformation begins with the embrace of love and leads to the first essential step, which is the transmutation of emotions. When you begin to tell yourself that your emotional stance in life is a distortion of your potential to love, then you have invited a flame into your life that will gradually destroy and transform you. (p. 20)

Life is synonymous with interaction. We are meant to be interactive beings: open, exchanging manifestations of a larger dimension, changing, disappearing, becoming manifest again.

To be open is to be vulnerable, an important characteristic of humanness. To be vulnerable is often to suffer. We tend to avoid suffering, and yet avoidance of suffering may deter movement to higher levels of consciousness. Suffering offers us the opportunity to transcend a particular situation.

Vaughan (1979) regards openness to experience as the hallmark of the healthy person. She addresses personal development in terms of the stages of identification and disidentification. In the identification stage the emphasis is on enhancing the self-image, raising self-esteem, and building ego strength. The stage of disidentification involves letting go of one's roles, possessions, activities, and relationships:

> Given a well established sense of authenticity and sound ego integration, individuals frequently come to psychotherapy plagued by a sense of meaninglessness and a feeling of apathy manifested as depression or, more acutely, as despair. Here the confrontation with death and aloneness and the first noble truth of Buddhism—that all life is suffering—are the predominant theme. (p. 27)

Successful resolution of this stage involves ego death; despair is transcended and awakening of transpersonal awareness occurs. At this level one feels a part of something larger than oneself:

> Transpersonal consciousness can be defined as that level of consciousness in which the underlying unity of all life is experientially realized as the ground of our being, and the universe itself is viewed as a dynamic web of relationships in continuous change. (p. 28)

Vaughan sees consciousness as the context of all experience: "the assumption here is that the more aware we are of the dynamics of our own being, the more we are capable of acting responsibly in the world" (p. 28). This statement corresponds to consciousness defined as the quality and diversity of interaction with the environment and also to Bentov's (1978) assertion that the higher the level of consciousness, the more control one has over the environment. Vaughan points out that shifting to consciousness as context facilitates disidentification and frees us from the domination of those things we identify with. All experiences are meaningful in the process of evolving consciousness.

Vulnerability, suffering, disease, death do not diminish us. What does diminish us is trying to protect ourselves by binding ourselves off from these experiences. The need is to let go, embrace our experience, and allow the expansion of consciousness to unfold.

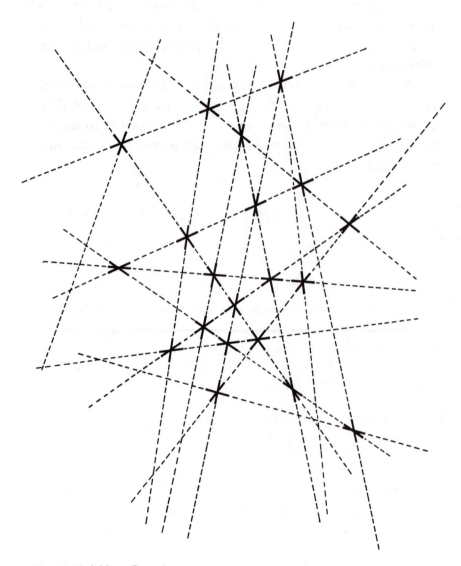

Fig. 18 Unfolding Consciousness

APPLICATION OF THE NEW PARADIGM OF HEALTH TO INDIVIDUALS, FAMILIES, AND COMMUNITIES

Joanne M. Marchione

Since its early beginnings nursing science has focused on the elaboration of relationships between persons and their environments relative to nursing, health, and illness. Nightingale (1859) conceptualized nursing as the science of health. She introduced persons, environments, and health as the basic concepts in need of nursing's consideration. Many interpretations of these concepts have evolved since the time of Nightingale. Various nurse theorists have chosen to place emphasis on one or more of these concepts in their formulation and development of nursing theory. Newman has chosen to elaborate a revolutionary concept of health as a new paradigm for health professionals. In this section I will discuss the meaning that this new paradigm of health has for clients. The word "client" is derived from the Latin word "cluo," which means "to hear." It is in its original sense of "mutual" hearing between the health professional and the client—as person, family, or community—that it is used here.

THE PARADOX OF UNIQUENESS
AND THE UNDIVIDED WHOLE

A paradigm of systems implies interconnectedness at every level. Persons, families, and communities are the human systems of concern to health professionals. These are the subjects and objects of concern that provide us with our reason to be. In viewing people as systems in interrelationships and in interconnection with each other, as well as connected with outside systems, we are able to focus on humans in holistic perspective:

> A paradigm of systems also implies (1) a redistribution, a recycling or energy interchange of all elements and structures, (2) a heterarchy or network of intercommunication, (3) complementarity of relationships to replace the dichotomous logic of previous mechanistic models, (4) uncertainty or probability and morphogenesis to replace static equilibrium of past models, and (5) change or transformation as a fundamental feature of self organizing living wholes. (Henderson, 1984–1985)

In this framework then, individuals, families, and communities are viewed as centers and fields of energy continually moving in dynamic interchange toward higher levels of expanding consciousness (Hanchett, 1979; Helvie, 1979, 1981; Newman, 1979, 1983b). As centers of energy each client system has a potential store of energy to act (Newman, 1979; Young, 1976a). As an energy field each client system represents an activated power source interpenetrating with other energy fields. For example, persons are continually interchanging energy with others "outside" themselves, families are in energy interchange with individuals and other families, communities with families, individuals, and other communities, and so forth. Thus client systems are interconnected in the sense that each is continually interchanging energy with the environment outside itself and with other client systems.

The underlying pattern of the whole of each person, family,

or community is considered the implicate order—the implicit representation of the whole (Bohm, 1980). The explicate order, that which is visable as part of the underlying whole, can be seen in explicit, observable patterns such as vortices of energy, networks of transfer of matter and information, and boundaries of space, time, and consciousness.

Hanchett (1979) refers to pattern as a static description of the dynamic energized structures we know as persons, families, or communities. This concept of pattern provides us with a stopgap picture, a freeze-frame view, a photographic representation of the whole of family or person or community. Just as the photograph or freeze-frame provides us with a partial view of the whole, with only a hint of what has gone before or what is to come, so in describing patterns of client systems we are provided a partial glimpse of the whole.

Client systems are "systematic wholes of self-regulating transformations . . . by which the parts of each are continually being articulated into an ever-changing whole" (Piaget, 1970, p. 44). This change or transformation is fundamental to the continual becoming of all human systems.

As systems, persons, families, and communities are organized as networks of relationships in interconnectedness. Networks are aggregates of connecting lines, links, and channels. The circulatory system of humans serves as a physiological example of a network as it provides for the distribution and redistribution of energies throughout the body. Likewise a family network includes a linkage of roles such as mother, wife, parent, daughter, housekeeper, financial provider, husband, lover, son, sibling. This same network expressed in social terms for community includes neighbors, friends, extended family members, teachers, ministers, employers, recreational leaders, transporters. Each of these linkages is interconnected by and through relationships. Each provides the environment of surrounding people for the other. Each of the client systems involves these interrelationships.

Interrelationships, viewed as movement or action, provide the pulse of client systems. The quality and quantity of energy interchanges manifested as patterned interrelationships provide the indexes for interpreting the health of persons or families or communities (Hanchett, 1979; Newman, 1979, 1983b).

Persons, families, and communities then cannot be dichotomized. They must be viewed as interconnected and relational, as undivided and whole. Bohm (1983) has noted that persons viewed as individuals are viewed as universal. He states:

> The individual is universal and the universal is the individual. The word "individual" means undivided . . . Individuality is only possible if it unfolds from wholeness. . . It is impossible to have true individuality except when grounded in the whole . . . Anything which is not in the whole is not individuality but egocentrism . . . The individual cannot be self centered . . . Anybody who is self-centered must be divided, because in order to become self-centered he must establish a division between himself and the whole . . . (p.35)

Rogers' (1970) concept of unitary man is embodied in this notion of universal/individual.

Families and communities are also undivided or individual and universal and yet continually in the process of transformation. Persons, families, and communities are seen in paradox, then, both as unique entities unto themselves and as persons or groups of persons in relationship with others. As Moustakas (1973) reminded us in his beautiful essay on creative life:

> Within every person is a distinct and unique being that is unlike any life that has existed before or will ever exist again. To maintain this uniqueness, when social and family pressures aim at suppressing or

destroying it, is the ultimate challenge of every human being. The unique person remains distinctive by exploring, discovering, continually unfolding in new ways and finding a sense of fulfillment in being rooted in life and creating new life . . . (p. 1)

This distinctive quality is also applicable for family and community.

NEWMAN'S CONCEPT OF HEALTH

In the early chapters of this text Newman explains health as a process. It is the "flow of life" seen as a kaleidoscopic evolution of patterning with paradoxes, contradictions, and ambiguities continually being synthesized into insights that lead to an ever-expanding consciousness. The revolutionary conceptualization of Newman's paradigm is the proposition that health is the synthesis of disease/nondisease. Newman's model embraces a dialectical outlook where transformation is basic, where the fundamental unit of analysis is movement, and where disease and nondisease are each reflections of a larger whole.

Transformation is conceptualized by Newman as expanding consciousness. Expanding consciousness occurs as a process of pattern recognition (insights) following a synthesis of contradictory events or disturbances in the flow of daily living. Pattern recognition is a spontaneous, sudden insight in relation to a shift in organizational complexity affording greater freedom and variety of responses to any given situation.

Movement provides an index for pattern recognition. Patterns of energy interchanging with events or environments and energy interchange through relationships with others constitute health. By relating with person(s) and event(s), no matter how instructive, constructive, or destructive some forces might seem to be, the energy of the event or other augments our own and gives us power to move through the particular situation. When we begin to see ourselves and others as centers of energy, we begin to grasp the pattern of the whole and can begin to think of ourselves and others as energy centers within an overall pattern of expanding consciousness.

Four variables are considered in interrelationship as critical linkages of the Newman paradigm. *Movement*, the manifestation of *consciousness*, is viewed in a complementary *space-time* relationship where time and space perceptions are useful as indications of health (expanding consciousness). Movement can be seen as waves of energy and energy transformation in the space and time of each of our lives.

PATTERNING OF INDIVIDUALS

The individual person is viewed here as a specific pattern of consciousness and yet at the same time an open energy field in interrelationship with others. Moustakas (1977) describes this paradox:

> The self exists as a whole with enduring presence and emerging patterns. Because of its uniqueness, depth and changing nature its qualities may be felt as reflections of an inconceivable totality or whole. The self of the individual may stand out in bold relief, or it may blend imperceptibly with other forms in nature and in the universe. It may be recognized through intuitive and unusual sense perceptions. (p. 2)

Personal insights are a mystery. One can participate in them, share them, live them in the existential sense, but they are often not explained by logic. Peck (1978) has suggested that the act of living (what he has called loving) requires a moving out—against the inertia of laziness through work and against the resistance engendered by fear—into the unknown and into the future. This moving out requires great risk and courage. This moving out, or growth, or expanded consciousness is often

painful as well as joyful. The process of expanding consciousness requires us to become aware of the value of suffering and
grief as well as of the value of joy and happiness. Each is a part
of our total being (Moustakas, 1977, p. 3; Peck, 1978, p. 133).

According to Jaspers (1963) the expanding consciousness
of self includes four formal characteristics: "(a) the feeling of
activity—an awareness of being active; (b) an awareness of
unity; (c) awareness of identity; and (d) awareness of the self
as distinct from an outer world and all that is not the self" (p.
21). Understanding of the paradox of consciousness and integration of self is again described in a passage from an earlier
work by Moustakas (1956):

> The self is itself alone existing as a totality and constantly emerging. It
> can be understood only as a unique person experience . . . True ex-
> perience may be understood through empathy in communal living. But
> it cannot be communicated. To communicate the self is to abstract from
> it, speak of its aspects or parts and then do violence to it. Communi-
> cation represents or symbolizes the self. (p. 3)

In the old paradigm, the highest level of development is
the development of the self, manifested in high self-esteem and
personal autonomy (Brandon, 1983). It incorporates feeling
good about one's self, feeling happy, lovable, and deserving.
Brandon claims that high self-esteem is based on the non-
conditional choice to seek or avoid awareness. He listed a variety of opposing issues relative to a person's volitional decision
to seek or avoid this awareness. Included among these issues
are (1) respect for reality versus avoidance of reality, (2) self-
confrontation versus self-avoidance, (3) receptivity to new
knowledge versus closed-mindedness, and (4) reason versus
irrationalism.

In the new paradigm, development proceeds beyond the
self into what Wilbur (1980) refers to as the mental-egoic realm,

a level at which the individual is more spontaneous than at the previous membership realm of self. At this level the emphasis is on unity with a greater whole and reconciliation of previously dichotomized states, such as love and hate, rationality and irrationality. Reconciling the earthy and the lofty in our lives is considered by Stone (1985) to be a constant requirement for personal involvement and cannot be done without interchange and relationship.

I propose that the issues raised by Brandon and Stone be viewed as complementary and indispensable antagonists occurring in a dialectical process by persons in their struggles toward higher levels of awareness. Self-confrontation and self-avoidance are two awareness issues with which we as selves are continually in the process of resolving. Both are necessary before we can move to higher levels of consciousness. It is often in the period of this struggle between self-confrontation and self-avoidance that insight occurs. A person may experience a long period of self-avoidance or self-confrontation or both before a higher level of awareness can be reached. I would further propose that relationship of self to self and self to other is often the catalyst for movement to a higher level of awareness. The insights required for these higher levels often require long periods of time and are often viewed as apparently acausal or multicausal. In other words, in our attempts to "know" ourselves as persons, we are continually resolving the desirable with the undesirable, the known with the unknown, the reasonable with the irrational.

Stone (1985) has addressed this issue of resolving paradoxes by use of the concept of the "disowned self." He suggests that the things we dislike are the representations of our disowned self (p. 71). Our disowned selves are quite unconscious to us, quite out of "awareness." Stone continues: "It is only as we become aware of all of our unconscious energy patterns that we can begin to exercise choice in our life and begin to take responsibility for what happens to us" (p. 98). "Every disowned energy pattern can work against us and can work against the evolution of consciousness" (p. 78). The process of evolving consciousness is facilitated by people becoming more fully aware of who they are, with full recognition and honor for all the living parts they discover in themselves (p. 126).

As Newman (1979, 1983b) and others (Dossey, 1982; Ferguson, 1980; Prigogine, 1980) have suggested, these struggles are the necessary "shakings up" or necessary disturbances that prevent stagnation and assist in the expansion of consciousness. Struggles or oppositional forces are catalysts for our transformation. The following case* serves as an example of this transformation:

> A client, Dana [fictitious name], is a divorcee with two preschool children, a 2-year-old boy and a girl aged 5. Her former spouse sometimes babysits with the children when Dana goes out for the evening. A brother who lives nearby is busy with a large family and two jobs. Dana and he visit only infrequently. Although her mother lives nearby, there is not a close relationship; her father lives in Texas and is not considered as part of her support system. She has a few "close friends" of long standing and is friendly with several other tenants in the apartment complex where she lives.
>
> Dana's economic support is generated by providing day care for a 9-month-old infant and three other preschool children. The infant is the son of one of her good friends. Her life is somewhat self-contained and routine.
>
> While under Dana's care, the 9-month-old infant died of sudden infant death syndrome (SIDS). The other children were present and

---

*This case study was obtained by personal communication with A. Kelly, nursing practitioner.

witnessed the event. Dana responded to the infant's death by administering cardiopulmonary resuscitation, for which she had received training. She notified the police, who took the baby to the hospital, and then notified the infant's family. She was able to get her mother-in-law to care for the other children while she joined the parents at the hospital.

A nurse interviewed Dana by phone shortly after the infant's death, offered her information about SIDS, and invited Dana to participate in a support group. The client requested additional information which would be appropriate for the children to assist them in understanding the event. She expressed uncertainty about responding to the "acting out" of the children.

When the nurse visited the home (by invitation of the client), Dana was crying and in a state of disorganization. The house was in disarray and two of the children were fighting; one of the children kept throwing toys at the mother. Dana complained of extreme fatigue and expressed a need to "be alone." She verbalized feelings of guilt despite having administered CPR to the baby. She spoke of being disinterested in her own children and frequently addressed them with irritation. She conveyed a sense of being quite overwhelmed by this experience. In addition, there were physical changes, including numerous "cold sores" around her mouth, and she complained of insomnia.

The nurse was able to assist Dana in reorganizing her situation. Dana expressed an interest in joining a support group and arranged with her mother-in-law to assist with the child care.

Fifteen weeks later the nurse revisited this client. Dana had been active in the support group over the last 15 weeks and had gained considerable comfort. In addition, she had received her instructor's license and was teaching a class on cardiopulmonary resuscitation. Other projects included helping to present a program for daycare providers about SIDS and arranging to have the county social service supply each licensed daycare provider with written information about SIDS. Most recently she had offered to serve on a local health services board in response to a newspaper announcement inviting such participation. Even so, she continued to cry when reminded of the death experience and displayed periods of sadness and remorse.

Following this event, Dana sees herself as more caring and sympathetic toward others, especially toward her children. She feels very close to her mother-in-law for the first time and her relationship with her ex-husband has improved. She has maintained a good relationship with the dead infant's parents and recently had dinner in their home.

The children freely discuss the death event and ask questions, which she feels comfortable in answering. She describes their behavior as "back to normal." The client explains that she is more outgoing now but expresses feelings of sadness and has stated that she will never get back to "normal."

Interpretation. Prior to the SIDS event the client was relatively isolated from adult family (spatial relationships), took little initiative to form meaningful relationships (movement), and was bored (perception of time). This pattern might be viewed as one of potential power and minimal energy interchange. It is characterized by a binding phase* in which everything was regulated and there was no need for initiative. With the experience of the sudden infant death, the "old rules" were no longer appropriate. Dana responded to this experience with self-consciousness and self-determination, *moving* into action and making appropriate choices, e.g., CPR, police, mother-in-law's assistance, support to the family in the hospital.

Following the event, her pattern was one of disorganization, manifested in her children's behavior, her home, and her feelings of not knowing what to do. In interaction with the nurse, she was able to utilize the power of the nurse's field of consciousness and began to reorganize her life in a more meaningful way. Her sadness itself was a more powerful emotion than the previous boredom. It is true that she will never return to her previous "normal" state, as she has had a transforming experience and is moving to another level of consciousness.

Once Dana began to work through this experience, first with disorganization and then with increased quality and quantity of interaction, a new awareness reflecting inner growth

---

*See also p. 44.

emerged. Dana's transcendence of the limitations of her previous situation has come with the emergence of a more complex level of interaction (time and movement) with her family and the community. In this way a greater range of environment (space) was available as both a resource and a recipient of energy transfer. Dana was able to learn the new "laws" of the situation and to move with them rather than against them. Her life reflected the increased quality and variety of her interaction.

PATTERNING OF FAMILIES

Families too are essentially dynamic processes, fields of energy and patterns of mirrored relationships that are not analyzable as separate parts. In searching for family health patterns, we seek to understand the whole. Kantor and Lehr (1975) have equated family patterns with strategies, or recurring patterns of interactional sequences, and continuous interchange of energies. Through awareness of such repetitions of sequence we begin to recognize typical movement patterns. These patterns evolve as members of a family act to regulate and shape the relationships between and among themselves. Persons joined together in an intimate relationship called family, whatever the bond, display patterns that are different from other groups.

Family health is defined by Newman (1983b) as the process of expanding consciousness of the family. Again, consciousness is defined as the informational capacity of the system and can be seen in the quantity and quality of interactions within the family and with the environment outside the family. In a family where there is a relatively high level of conciousness, there is a high level of spontaneity. Members are not locked into rigid responses, either to each other or to stimuli from outside the family. The easy flow of energy within and outside the family facilitates further and continuous expansion of consciousness.

Spontaneity is an important variable in family health. Lewis, et. al. (1976, p. 103) describe healthy families as those who are open to many possibilities and who are continually operating with several strategies for maintaining family life. Also included in the characteristics of healthy families are those who demonstrate the ability to have meaningful relationships and encounters in the broader environment outside the family. Family relationships that reach into the wider community are sources of stimulation that add life to the family system. This point is consistent with the premise that in order for a system to grow, it must use energy from the environment (Von Bertalanffy, 1968).

Other family theorists have also noted the importance of interactive patterns within and outside the family. Reiss and Oliveri (1980) consider the following characteristics as important to health in families: employing a problem-solving style that includes a cooperative, effective search for family patterns, a shared perception of trust in each other as family members, and a trusting perception of the social world outside the family Pratt's (1976) study of family interaction led her to describe an energized family as one who manifests high interactions within and outside the family.

Central to the theory of family health as expanding consciousness is the premise that disease within the family is to be considered a manifestation of the family pattern and as such understood as a possible factor in family integration and transformation. If one or more family members' becoming ill is the only way the family can become conscious of itself, then that is health in process for that family. This approach to family study posits a synthesized view of opposing forces, in this case disease and nondisease, in a meaningful pattern of the health (life) process (Newman, 1983b).

Stanton (1984), a family theorist, also subscribes to this synthesized view to explain patterns of health in families. He has described members of a family system as continually engaging in a two-faceted process of approaching and retreating. Specifically, the family is continually in the process of oscillating between the thesis of approaching and the antithesis of retreating toward eventual synthesis or transcendance of this seeming dichotomy to achieve a balance of distance regulation (Kantor & Lehr, 1975). The reality of this distance regulation is not only the one (approaching) nor the other (retreating) but the process of continual movement between these poles. Stanton has stressed the importance of recognizing the coexistence of opposites within family systems where individual family members may continue to move in their own patterned spheres while also contributing to the choreographic whole of the family. At the same time the family as a unit may also be moving in a similar pattern relative to different demands and features of its context.

Piaget (1970) cautioned that an adequate understanding of structures (patterns) cannot be reduced to an understanding of the properties of parts. What is primary is the self-regulating transformations by which the parts are continually being articulated into an ever-changing whole.

Piaget's primary emphasis on transformation is echoed by Doherty's approach to the study of family (Doherty, 1984). Doherty urges investigators to focus on family events rather than things. Viewed in this way, families are seen as having elements of identity-forming permanence and of transforming change. Awareness of events and processes helps to avoid focusing on the permanent features ascribed to families and promotes a recognition of the emergent features, here considered evolving patterns of consciousness.

Doherty (1984) has advocated the use of complementary theories as the most enriching approach to the understanding of family phenomena. For example, one time the focus of assessment might be on the overt family movement patterns and the next time on the meaning these patterns hold for family members; one time assessing the family as influenced by the larger social context of church, school, and workplace, and the next time looking at the family as influencing these same factors. With this approach knowledge of family takes into account counterbalancing perspectives.

Kantor and Lehr (1975) have described families in relationships among themselves and between the family and persons outside the family. Families change and respond productively to strain, tension, and stress—the inevitable and necessary consequences of their interchange with the world outside the family. Through their information processing capacity families are able to elaborate and/or change their action patterns. This information processing requires a shift away from the flow of energy required by the individual members of the family in order to interrelate and transmit information. Families seek to attain their goals by continually informing their members what constitutes an optimal distance, as relationships among members in the context of specific events become established and fluctuate. The predominant feature of a family's information process is the communication process which, in open family systems, becomes more and more fluid.

Kantor and Lehr have suggested that a general pattern of accumulation and expenditure of energy is common to all families. It is through the recording of this energy flow that one can determine whether or not a family has enough energy to meet its demands or enough energy demands to utilize its supply. By detecting these energy patterns one is able to identify the intensity of family experience. Energy patterns are equated with family movement or activity.

Movement patterns in family are the visible manifestations of the interconnectedness of its members, a fundamental aspect of the family's social organization. The shared movements of work and play, of loving and fighting, are nowhere more evident than in family relationships. Movement is an indicator of family health and has been described in terms of spatial shifts among family members and shifts in the interface between the family and external systems such as friendship networks, neighborhood, and health care professionals (Stanton, 1984).

A multiplicity of patterned moves are available to a family. Kantor and Lehr (1975) have identified three basic forms of patterning: (1) maintenance patterns—those concerned with preserving the family relationships as they are; (2) stress patterns—those concerned with accentuating and accelerating the natural tensions among family members, occasionally pushing the family's relationships into confusion and turmoil; and (3) repair patterns—those concerned with modifying activities that keep the family viable. This patterning sequence is much like that described by Hall and Cobey (1974). They have noted that the rhythm of the perceived world is constantly changing and that people go through phases of preparation, characterized by confusion (stress patterns); action, characterized by mastery of movement and a capacity for balance (maintenance); and recovery or reorientation, clarity of organization, and ease of movement (repair).

A pattern of enablement has also been identified by Kantor and Lehr (1975) as indicative of the healthy family. An enabling pattern is defined as one where families maintain a distance regulation balance, that is, an ability to recognize and affirm differences so that no member is consistently or systematically denied actualization of goals. Inflexibility or rigidity in family patterning and inability to recognize or affirm differences, along with an authoritarian style of governing, are the most visible features of family disablement. Pratt (1976) had also identified healthy families as energized families with patterns of enablement. She characterized the healthy, energized family as one in which family process includes an egalitarian governance with shared power, autonomy, and freedom of movement for individual family members.

Kantor and Lehr (1975) have further described three major patterns of family systems. In the open family system order and change are expected to result from the interactions of relatively stable, evolving family structures (movable space, variable time, and flexible energy). Patterns of enablement are most evident in open family systems. In closed family systems stable structures (fixed space, regular time, and steady energy) are relied upon as reference points for order and change. Random family systems are characterized as unstable structures (dispersed space, irregular time, and fluctuating energy) experimented with as a reference point for order and change. Patterns of disablement are frequently seen in closed and random family systems.

Fluctuating, rhythmic patterns of enablement/disablement occur as families are able to synthesize issues related to distance regulation. Family members are constantly concerned with questions of spatial closeness-distance, with joining-separating issues, with congruent-incongruent issues of dates and time, and with issues related to freedom of movement within and outside the family.

Since Newman endorses the basic assumption of the living system as an open system, the categories of family patterns suggested by Kantor and Lehr—open, closed, and random— are not to be interpreted literally. The family labeled a "closed system" is an open system but manifests itself in more fixed, regular, and certain patterns of relating than the "open system" family. Newman has suggested that one might consider the "random system" as a representation of points of disorganization/reorganization of the family. The fluctuating distance regulation patterns characteristic of these types are viewed from the perspective of Newman's model as efforts of the system to reorganize at a higher level. Families may move through all three types in the course of their evolution. However, according to Kantor and Lehr, a predominant family pattern may emerge.

The following family case is one example from a larger study of families with different situations that required altered mobility (any change in the activity patterns among family members). This case illustrates the emergence of a pattern of expanding consciousness when a new member with divergent movement patterns was temporarily added to the family unit. The quality and quantity of interactions were deduced from the descriptions obtained from family members as they described the event and their responses to it. (All names have been changed to protect identity.) These responses were referenced in time and space and were manifested as movement and consciousness.

Mrs. Scott, a part-time secondary school teacher, her husband, a sales representative in a textile firm, their two children, Claudia, age seven years, and Jeremy, age eleven years, and Sammie, a two-year-old Collie dog, share a small home in suburbia. Mr. Atlas, a friend who had lost his home in a recent divorce settlement, was invited to stay with the family for three weeks until he was able to locate a residence of his own. He was also a senior supervisor of Mr. Scott. Mr. Atlas delayed his search for housing and extended his stay with the Scott family for six months. This addition to the Scott household was perceived by all family members as a transforming event requiring alterations of time, space, and movement patterns.

Space. The Scott family lived in a modestly furnished, three-bedroom ranch-style home in a middle-class suburban neighborhood. Because each of the bedrooms was occupied, Mr. Atlas was given the family room, separated from the master bedroom only by a small bath. The family room had been a place for shared and coordinated activities for the family before Mr. Atlas's arrival. For instance, games were played here, craft projects were accomplished, and television programs were viewed together since this was the location of the family's only television set. The family room space was now regarded as the "territory" of Mr. Atlas, and all members of the Scott family were cautious in their use of the room when he was not occupying it [or conscious of not being able to carry out their usual activities]. The children described how they had to wait until Mr. Atlas moved out of the room each Saturday morning so they could watch their favorite cartoons. Mrs. Scott was often unable to do her needlework because Mr. Atlas frequently occupied the chair in the family room with the best lighting, one that she had used for needlework prior to his visit.

Mr. Atlas had a different view of personal space than was the pattern for the Scott family. He liked to hug and kiss each of the Scott family members when coming and going. Mrs. Scott was uncomfortable with this practice and explained that she and her husband had not been socialized to use these gestures with others outside the family. Even though she had apprised Mr. Atlas of this preference, he continued the practice, dismissing their reluctances as a stereotypical pattern of their ethnicity: "Their kind" conveyed an attitude of "distance and cold" while his "people" were "warmer and closer." Mrs. Scott acknowledged that she and her family had become somewhat more appreciative of alternative modes of expressing affection since Mr. Atlas's visit.

Time. Until Mr. Atlas arrived, the family dinner ritual was approximately one hour. During this time the family shared the preparation and cleaning activities associated with dinner, and their discussions at mealtime usually included a sharing of their day's events. Meal times were also used to discuss immediate or long-term goals of individual members and/or specific family goals. After Mr. Atlas arrived, the dinner ritual was extended to four hours to accommodate his preference for before and after dinner drinks, fine wines, and gourmet dining. He often spoke of showing the Scott family an improved lifestyle. The dinner conversations also shifted from present/future orientations to reviews of the past childhoods of Mr. Atlas and Mr. and Mrs. Scott.

Private and coordinated times were greatly diminished due to the long hours spent with the dinner ritual. Also, Mr. Atlas disregarded the time the family needed for private and shared activities. Once when Mr. Atlas was invited to attend one of Jeremy's sports events, he remarked: "Isn't it too bad that everyone has to be manipulated by Jeremy just because he wants to engage in sports?" Eventually, however, Mr. Atlas agreed to participate in these family spectator events.

Movement. Shared and coordinated movements were greatly diminished due to the prolonged dinner rituals and the constrained family room space. Prior to Mr. Atlas's arrival all household activities, including washing, ironing, cleaning, and cooking, were shared. Wanting to please her husband's friend (and boss) in the early days of his visit, and because Mr. Atlas had expressed the belief that household activities were the responsibilities of a "good wife and mother," Mrs. Scott soon assumed all of these activities alone. Private interests, such as yoga classes and excursions with friends, were sharply diminished. Finding these restrictions untenable after a few months, Mrs. Scott began to reassert herself and convinced Mr. Scott that a modified version of their previous pattern of shared activities was much more equitable and satisfying. They redefined the shared activities and attempted to include Mr. Atlas in the redistribution of household chores.

Mr. and Mrs. Scott's sexual relations were curtailed. They described their reluctance to move about freely in their bedroom because they were aware that sounds carried to and from the family room via the bathroom plumbing fixtures.

Mr. Scott's movement outside the family was also curtailed. Prior to Mr. Atlas's arrival, Mr. Scott had played handball two nights a week with friends at a nearby racquet club. On alternating evenings he accompanied his wife to their children's ball games or dance classes. Now his time was spent mostly "entertaining" Mr. Atlas in the long dinner ritual at home. Mr. Scott often fell asleep in the evenings when the conversation waned. Prior to Mr. Atlas's visit, Mr. Scott had been working to reduce his hypertension by modifying his dietary patterns and had stopped smoking. With the altered dining rituals and limitations of activity within and outside the family, he reverted to his previous patterns.

The family dog's activities were also altered during Mr. Atlas's visit. He had insisted that the dog had not been adequately trained and took over this activity by issuing various commands to the dog each evening before dinner. Prior to Mr. Atlas's arrival, each of the family members had shared in the training of the dog, but the bulk of the training had been done by Mrs. Scott.

The choice point. Mr. and Mrs. Scott became aware of their loss of power in the distribution of shared activities. As previously described, they acted on this awareness by improving the quality of their interactions through a reorganization of their movement patterns. Jeremy became aware of a lack of access to his father. He began to ask when he could see his father alone, for play time and decision making, as they had done in the past. He also began to consult with his mother and sister on personal decision making. The dog began to resist the rigorous exercise Mr. Atlas was asking him to do. He eventually rolled over and urinated on the carpet when Mr. Atlas issued his commands. This action effectively extinguished Mr. Atlas's training program. Claudia's needs and goals as an equal person in the family became more apparent as she began to be more assertive during Mr. Atlas's visit. Mr. and Mrs. Scott described a new regard for her contributions in family decision making.

As the Scott family began to assert themselves, the restrictions of space, time, and movement imposed by Mr. Atlas's presence were gradually released. The dinner time was reduced to one hour with shared distribution of activities redefined and reorganized. Territory in the family room, other than during the time when Mr. Atlas was sleeping, was gradually redefined for shared and coordinated family activities.

Six months passed, and Mr. Atlas, who no longer viewed himself as a visitor but as a family member, announced that he would stay for another six months. Finding this decision unacceptable, Mr. and Mrs. Scott developed strategies for moving him out of their home. At first they suggested that he needed his privacy. When this strategy failed, they told him that they needed to rediscover theirs. They expressed their feelings about their losses of shared and coordinated family space-time. They helped him find an apartment by sharing newspaper ads of potential apartments with him each day. The relationship with Mr. Atlas was maintained and strengthened after his move out of the home, as was evidenced by the family's frequent inclusion of him in family events.

Interpretation. The Scott family reached a new level of consciousness by their ability to recognize and refine their interaction patterns. Mr. Atlas's demands could be viewed as a disturbing, tension-producing event, a perturbation in the life of the Scott family. The evolution of consciousness often requires a "shaking up," a disturbance. According to Prigogine (1980), humans who are insulated from disturbance are protected from necessary developmental change. Disturbances such as those described in the Scott family are a part of the developmental process of the family.

Mr. Scott's ability to assert himself as the head of the household was cited as one of the most important "redeeming qualities" of this transforming event. The family expressed a renewed enjoyment of shared relationships.

Patterns are not always this easily discernible. As Laing (1969) so aptly pointed out: "We ourselves, all of us, are ourselves the elements of the patterns we are trying to discern." Person and family patterns "are not laid out before us like the stars in the sky" (p. 86). Each of us is "acting parts in a play that we have never read and never seen, whose plot we don't know, whose existence we can glimpse, but whose beginning and end are beyond our present imagination and conception" (p. 87).

Discovery of a new pattern transcends expectations (Ferguson, 1980). Shifting from an old to a new pattern is qualitatively sudden, whereby the seeing of pattern is not sequential but all at once. This shift in awareness is an "awakening, liberating, unifying and transforming" experience (Ferguson, 1980). Pattern can often be seen but not always comprehended by an "outsider," i.e., one without experience to know what to look for in a given situation. Experience is the transformation of preconceived notions and expectations by means of repeated encounters with actual situations. It implies that there is a dialogue between what is observed and what is expected (Benner & Wrubel, 1982). It is through the awareness of such repetitions of sequence that one usually begins to recognize typical family movement patterns (Kantor & Lehr, 1975). Only when the sequence of movements or the relationship of acts is perceived can the overall pattern itself be known (Capra, 1982; Stulman, 1972).

PATTERNING OF COMMUNITIES

The concept of "community" is discussed here in its relational sense, as described by Gusfield (1975). In this sense community is perceived as a characteristic of human relationships where group members are interchanging energies in an ever-evolving "dance" of cooperation and conflict. These relationships provide the meaning of community for all of us as individuals (Hanchett, 1979).

The act of our relating in a shared situation as two or more energy fields in search of common goals provides a sense of community. A community consists of four basic elements—people, place, resources and services, and the relationships between the people and between the people, the place, and the resources (Hanchett, 1979). These relationships are a reflection of the health or expanding consciousness of community. Also, the community of our past, present, and future is mirrored in our relationships with others. This notion of the sensing of the whole of our being as community in a timeless act is addressed by Gendlin (1973) in the following passage:

> Going through a simple act involves an enormous number of familiarities, learnings, senses for the situation, understanding of life and people, as well as the many specifics of a given situation. All this goes into just saying "hello" in a fitting way to a not very close friend . . . The feel of doing anything involves our sense of the whole situation at any moment, despite our focally reflecting on it as such. (p. 370)

The recurrent and explicit actions of our relating with others provide us "as a community" as well as outsiders with a view of the patterns of the whole situation at any moment. In Bohm's (1983) terms, then, the actions of relating are explicit representations that provide a glimpse of the whole of our implicit worlds. The whole of our world, how we see ourselves and others within the context of community, is reflected in our acts of relating. These acts of relating reveal patterns of movement and consciousness.

Community is founded upon people, conceived in their wholeness, and linked to identity of common interests, to a sense of belonging, to shared cultural and ethnic ideas and values, and to a way of life (Plant, 1974). People as "community" are inextricably linked to each other through various patterns of relating (Hanchett, 1979).

Community members are characterized as organized energy fields, linked together as a unit by interdependence and interaction to accomplish group goals (Helvie, 1979, 1981). Kinetic energy (movement) in community systems relates to who does what, who is accountable to whom, and other role activities, as well as the overt and covert rules about movement within and outside the unit. Potential energy refers to the available energy manifested in the knowledge, attitudes, skills, physical stamina, flexibility, and cohesiveness of community members for meeting the changing needs of the group and evolving through stages of development and situational crises that occur.

From the standpoint of energy interchange, movement (interaction) is a powerful indicator of community consciousness, referenced in space and time of community members individually and collectively. If we can discover the field of experiences, expressed in relationships, and seen as encompassing movement-space-time patterns of a particular community, we can discover the context in which members of that community interpret their world.

In a classic work, *Health, Culture and Community*, Paul (1955) suggested the search for patterning of culture as an organizing framework for understanding the whole that makes up the life of a community and as a means whereby the health care professional can learn to view health from the standpoint of the person(s) in a community. People live in an environment of climate, terrain, and natural resources, as well as one of a kind of collective consciousness called culture. Culture reveals the transformation of a community's habitat, in the form of tunnels and towers, a particular form of clothes, response to environmental pollutants, and so on. People also interpret their environment according to rules implicit in the prevailing culture. Relationships are reflected in culture. Culture can be viewed as the consciousness of community.

The health of the community, viewed in terms of the quality and quantity of interactions within the community and between the community and the environment, is a reflection of the total design. Background patterns of a community will scarcely appear spontaneously to the one who fixes attention exclusively on foreground phenomena (Paul, 1955). Gusfield (1975) stressed the importance of viewing the concept of community as a dimension of an influential, pervasive, and significant contrast. Community is to be viewed with its counterconcepts— individual, family, society—and examined in light of the synthesis and symbiosis of these patterns. Paired concepts, such as individual and community or family and community, when viewed together reveal relationships that, while pointing in opposite directions, are inextricably linked.

Goeppinger, Lassiter, and Wilcox (1982) have described community health as the ability of a community and its constituents to interact effectively, that is, to construct and utilize structures that allow people in a community to manage the problems of their collective life while at the same time encouraging its members to lead satisfying and productive lives. Community health is defined as self-awareness, a means of communicating and a source of control of environment—i.e., expanding consciousness. The interaction, action, and awareness categories of the unitary pattern assessment framework developed by a group of nurse theorists (Roy et al., 1982) are consistent with this definition of community health.

The East Central Ohio tornado experience in the spring of 1985 serves to illustrate the expanding consciousness of community. The quality and quantity of interactions (energy interchanges) of members from within and people outside the community were increased considerably as a result of the environmental disaster. Many of those who lost their homes were "taken in" by neighbors and relatives, some even by strangers who simply wanted to give of their services to aid the destitute. A network of support systems evolved.

The National Guard was mobilized by the governor for restoration of order and to protect the remains of property from looting. The local and nearby Red Cross agencies brought volunteer assistance, medical supplies, food, and clothing. The

Boy Scouts of America volunteered to help local and surrounding firemen clear the debris. The Scouts also brought food, clothing, and toys for the children. Nearby industry, such as General Electric, offered a job-sharing program for those who were left jobless by the destruction and closing of their companies. Surrounding schools and churches offered shelter and solace; hospitals and health care professionals provided medical and often free/voluntary health care; and so on (see, for example, *Time Magazine*, June 3, 1985).

The "community" expanded to new vistas when nearby neighbors, industries, and organizations lent their support and assistance to rebuild the small city. New relationships were formed and old ones strengthened or transformed by this chaotic natural event.

The community was soon compared with a city in the western portion of the state that had been nearly destroyed by a similar tornado only 11 years before. Hopes were kept high by the example of the city to the west, which had realized numerous improvements as a result of the rebuilding and reconstruction following the destruction of the tornado. People in the East Central Ohio town began to take an active role in the planning for the rebuilding of their recently devastated city. A new sense of "community" was evident among many people of disparate socioeconomic, ethnic, and educational statuses, who came together for the common goal of rebuilding their city. Many new networks evolved.

Interpretation. This "community," once a quiet, self-sufficient, almost isolated, dispersed group of people, evolved and expanded as a result of the common experience of the tornado. The tornado might be thought of as a giant fluctuation that moved the community to a deeper sense of life's meanings and to recognize the value and importance of relationships.

Transformations in this community occurred on many levels. Members of the community were reenergized by the mutual experience of this disastrous event. Internal and external relationships were strengthened and expanded. A new, expanded sense of "community" was emerging. This was truly an example of the expanding consciousness of community.

The threads of personal, family, and community health are woven into the sociocultural fabric of "community." These threads are visible through relationships—relationships of persons to themselves, persons to family, and persons to community. Threads, here described as patterns of energy interchange, within and outside person, family, and community systems, provide the indexes for measuring the health of a people.

RESPONSIBILITY OF HEALTH PROFESSIONALS

As health professionals, we have only to look at the patterning of relationships among people to discern their expanding consciousness. The quality of our relationships as health professionals with clients who seek our assistance and care is critical. Moustakas (1977) described genuine relating as a "process of intuitive awareness, sensing and knowing—a recognition of the mystery and awe, the capriciousness and unpredictability of life." He advised us to become aware of the power of silence and of real dialogue with others in the "deep moments of life" (p. 13). As a professional in relationships with people, families, and communities, I have become increasingly aware of the significance of our interactions and the unpredictable, mysterious, sometimes spiritual quality of our energy interchange via these relationships.

BIBLIOGRAPHY

Abse, D.W., Wilkins, M.M., VandeCastle, R.L., Buxton, W.D., Demars, J.B., Brown, R.S., & Kirschoner, L.G. (1974). Personality and behavioral characteristics of lung cancer patients. *Journal of Psychosomatic Research, 18,* 101–113.

Ainsworth-Land, G. (1984). *New rules for growth and change.* Eden Prairie, MN: Wilson Learning Corp.

Ainsworth-Land, G. & V. (1982). *Forward to basics.* Buffalo, NY: D.O.K.

Allport, G. (1961). *Pattern and growth in personality.* New York: Holt, Rinehart & Winston.

Ardell, D.B. (1977). *High level wellness.* Emmaus, PA: Rodale Press.

Bathrop, R.W. (1977). Depressed lymphocyte function after bereavement. *Lancet, 16*(4), 834–836.

Behnke, E.A. (1974). Space-time concepts as world-dimensions. *Main Currents, 31*(1), 13–17.

Benner, P., & Wrubel, J. (1982). Skilled clinical knowledge: the value of perceptual awareness, parts I and II, *The Journal of Nursing Administration, 5* (1), 42–48; *6,* 28–33.

Bentov, I. (1978). *Stalking the wild pendulum.* New York: E. P. Dutton.

Blake, M.J.F. (1967). Relationship between circadian rhythm of body temperature and introversion-extroversion. *Nature, 215,* 896–897.

Bohm, D. (1980). *Wholeness and the implicate order.* London: Routledge & Kegan Paul.

Bohm, D. (1981). The physicist and the mystic—is a dialogue between them possible? A conversation with David Bohm conducted by Renee Weber. *Re-Vision, 4*(1), 22–35.

Bohm, D. (1983). Of matter and meaning: the super implicate order. A conversation between David Bohm and Renee Weber. *Re-Vision, 6*(1), 34–44.

Brandon, N. (1983). *Honoring the self: personal integrity and the heroic potentials.* Los Angeles: J. P. Tarcher.

Brent, S.B. (1978). Prigogine's model for self-organization in nonequilibrium systems: its relevance for developmental psychology. *Human Development, 21,* 374–387.

Capra, F. (1982). *The turning point.* New York: Simon & Schuster.

Cassandra. (1983). Membership bulletin. (P.O. Box 341, Williamsville, NY 14221)

Chetanananda, S. (1985). The symphony of life. *The American Theosophist*, *73*(5), 152–174.

Colquhoun, W.P. (1971). Circadian variations in mental efficiency. In W.P. Colquhoun (Ed.). *Biological rhythms and human performance*. New York: Academic Press, pp. 39–107.

Condon, W.S. (1980). The relation of interactional synchrony and cognitive and emotional processes. In M.R. Key (Ed.). *The relationship of verbal and nonverbal communication*. New York: Moutin Publishing, pp. 48–65.

Davis, M. (1982). *Interaction rhythms: periodicity in communicative behavior*. New York: Human Sciences.

DeLong, A.J. (1981). Phenomenological space-time: toward an experiential relativity. *Science*, *213*(7), 681–683.

DeLong, A.J., & Lubar, J.F. (1979). Effect of environmental scale of subjects on spectral EEG output. *Society for Neuroscience Abstracts*, *5*, 203.

Dembroski, T.M., MacDougall, J.M., Eliot, R.S., & Buell, J.C. (1984). Moving beyond Type A. *Advances*, *1*(1), 16–25.

Doberneck, B. (1985). Personal communication. May 1.

Doherty, W. (1984). *Quanta, quarks and families: implications of modern physics*. Paper presented at the Theory and Methods Workshop, National Council on Family Relations, San Francisco.

Dolfman, M.L. (1973). The concept of health: an historic and analytic examination. *Journal of School Health*, *43*, 491–497.

Dossey, L. (1982). *Space, time, and medicine*. Boulder: Shambhala.

Dossey, L. (1984). *Beyond illness: discovering the experience of health*. Boulder: Shambhala.

Dubos, R. (1965). *Man adapting*. New Haven, CT: Yale University Press.

Dunn, H.L. (1959). High-level wellness for man and society. *American Journal of Public Health*, *49*, 786–792.

Dunn, H.L. (1973). *High level wellness*. Arlington, VA: Beatty.

Ferguson, M. (1980). *The aquarian conspiracy: personal and social transformation in the 1980's*. Los Angeles: J.P. Tarcher.

Friedman, H. L. (1983). The self-expansiveness level form: a conceptualization and measurement of a transpersonal construct. *The Journal of Transpersonal Psychology*, *15*, November 1, 37–50.

Friedman, M., & Rosenman, R.H. (1974). *Type A behavior and your heart*. New York: Alfred A. Knopf.

Fuller, R.B. (1975). *Synergetics*. New York: Macmillan Inc.

Gendlin, E.T. (1973). A phenomenology of emotion: anger. In D. Carr & E. Casey (Eds.). *Explorations in phenomenology*. The Hague: Martinus: Nijhoff.

Gendlin, E.T. (1978). *Focusing*. New York: Everest.

Goeppinger, J., Lassiter, P., & Wilcox, B. (1982). Community health is community competence. *Nursing Outlook*, September-October, 464–467.

Gottlieb, R. (1982). Vision training provides window to brain change. *Brain-Mind Bulletin*, 7(17), 1–2.

Gottlieb, R. (1983). *The eye gym and the power to know*. Power of Knowing Conference, Berkeley, CA, May 25–27.

Gusfield, J. (1975). *Community: a critical response*. New York: Harper & Row.

Hall, E.T. (1959). *The silent language*. Greenwich, CT: Fawcett.

Hall, E.T. (1984). *The dance of life: the other dimension of time*. Garden City, NY: Anchor/Doubleday.

Hall, R. L., & Cobey, V.E. (1974). The world as crystallized movement. *Main Currents*, 31(1), 4–7.

Hanchett, E. (1979). *Community health assessment: a conceptual tool kit*. New York: John Wiley & Sons.

Hart, L.A. (1978). The new "brain" concept of learning. *Phi Delta Kappan*, February, 393–396.

Helvie, C.O. (1979). A proposed theory for nursing in community health, Parts I and II. *Canadian Journal of Public Health*, 70, January/February, 41–46; July/August, 266–270.

Helvie, C.O. (1981). *Community health nursing: theory and process*. New York: Harper & Row.

Henderson, H. (1984–1985). Post economic policies for post industrial society. *Re-Vision*, 7(2), 20–29.

Heron, J. (1981). Philosophical basis for a new paradigm. In P. Reason & J. Rowan (Eds.). *Human inquiry: a sourcebook of new paradigm research*. New York: John Wiley & Sons, pp. 19–35.

Hofstadter, D.R. (1979). *Godel, Escher, Bach: an eternal golden braid*. New York: Vintage.

Jantsch, E. (1980). *The self-organizing universe*. New York: Pergamon Press.

Jaspers, K. (1957) *General psychopathology*. Manchester, England: Manchester University Press.

Jaspers, K. (1963). *Man in the modern age*. New York: Doubleday.

Jones, R.S. (1982). *Physics as metaphor*. New York: Meridian.

Kallio, J.T. (1979). *The relationship among perceived control, mood states, and perception of nursing care for a control-induced and comparison group of patients in the critical care setting*. Unpublished master's thesis, University of Minnesota, Minneapolis.

Kane, C. (1985). The clovers connection. *Cassandra: Radical Feminist Nurses' Newsjournal, 3*(1), 21–22.

Kantor, D., & Lehr, W. (1975). *Inside the family*. New York: Harper Colophon.

Kaufman, M.A. (1969). A time, stress, perception model for theory development. *Proceedings of the First Nursing Theory·Conference*. Kansas City: University of Kansas Medical Center Department of Nursing Education, pp. 23–32.

Keen, S. (1978). Self-love and the cosmic connection. *Re-Vision, 1*(3/4), 88–89.

Kleitman, N. (1963). *Sleep and wakefulness*. Chicago: University of Chicago Press.

Krieger, D. (1979). *The therapeutic touch: how to use your hands help or heal*. Englewood Cliffs, NJ: Prentice-Hall.

Krippner, S. (Ed.) (1973). *Galaxies of life*. New York: Interface.

Kunz, D., & Peper, E. (1982–1983). Fields and their clinical implications, Parts I and II. *The American Theosophist*.

Laing, R.D. (1969). *The politics of the family*. New York: Pantheon.

Land, G.T.L. (1973). *Grow or die*. New York: Dell.

Leonard, G. (1978). *The silent pulse*. New York: E. P. Dutton.

Lerner, M. and Remen, R.N. (1985). Varieties of integral cancer therapies. *Advances, 2*(3), 14–33.

LeShan, L. (1966). An emotional life-history pattern associated with neoplastic disease. *Annals of the New York Academy of Science, 125,* 780–793.

LeShan, L. (1977). *You can fight for your life*. New York: M. Evans.

Lewis, J., Beavers, W. R., Gossett, J. R., & Phillips, V. A. (1976). *No single thread: psychological health in family systems*. New York: Bruner/Mazel.

Manthey, M. (1980). *The practice of primary nursing*. Boston: Blackwell Scientific.

Manthey, M. (1985). Paper presented at a Conference of Nurse Executives, University of Minnesota, Minneapolis, MN.

Masson, V. (1985). Nurses and doctors as healers. *Nursing Outlook, 33*(2), 70–73.

Mikunas, A. (1974). The primacy of movement. *Main Currents, 31*(1), 8–12.

Minors, D.S., & Waterhouse, J.M. (1984). The sleep-wakefulness rhythm, exogenous and endogenous factors (in man). *Experientia, 40,* 410–416.

Minuchin, S., Rossman, B., & Baker, L. (1978). *Psychosomatic families—Anorexia nervosa in context*. Cambridge: Harvard University Press.

Moss, R. (1981). *The I that is we*. Millbrae, CA: Celestial Arts.

Moustakas, C.F. (Ed.) (1956). *The self explorations in personal growth*. New York: Harper & Row.

Moustakas, C.F. (1977). *Creative life*. New York: Van Nostrand, Reinhold.

Murdoch, E.B., & Kenedi, R.M. (1981). Patterning of human body movement in and through space. *Physiotherapy, 67*, 35–37.

Muses, C. (1978). *Higher dimensions and systems relating science and spirit.* Paper presented at symposium on New Dimensions of Consciousness, sponsored by Sufi Order in the West, New York, November 17–20.

Nemeth, I., & Meezi, M. (1967). Cancer and psychological factors in a select sample. *Journal of Psychosomatic Research, 12*, 55–60.

Newman, M.A. (1972). Time estimation in relation to gait tempo. *Perceptual and Motor Skills, 34*, 359–366.

Newman, M.A. (1976). Movement tempo and the experience of time. *Nursing Research, 25*, 273–279.

Newman, M.A. (1979). *Theory development in nursing.* Philadelphia: F.A. Davis.

Newman, M.A. (1982). Time as an index of expanding consciousness with age. *Nursing Research, 31*, 290–293.

Newman, M.A. (1983a). Editorial. *Advances in Nursing Science, 5*(2), x–xi.

Newman, M.A. (1983b). Newman's health theory. In I. Clements & F. Roberts (Eds.). *Family health: a theoretical approach to nursing care.* New York: John Wiley & Sons, pp. 161–175.

Newman, M.A. (1984). Nursing diagnosis: looking at the whole. *American Journal of Nursing, 84*, 1496–1499.

Newman, M.A. (1986). Nursing's emerging paradigm: the diagnosis of pattern. In A. Maclean (Ed.). *Lecture notes on clinical medicine.* St. Louis: The C.V. Mosby Co.

Nightingale, F. (1859). *Notes on nursing: what it is and what is not.* New York: Dover.

Ostrander, S., & Schroeder, L. (1971). *Psychic discoveries behind the iron curtain.* New York: Bantam Books.

Parsons, T. (1958). Definitions of health and illness in the light of American values and social structure. In E. Jaco (Ed.). *Patients, physicians, and illness.* Glencoe, IL: Free Press.

Paul, B. (Ed.) (1955). *Health, culture and community.* New York: Russell Sage Foundation.

Peck, M.S. (1978). *The road less travelled.* New York: Simon & Schuster.

Peck, M.S. (1983). *People of the lie.* New York: Simon & Schuster.

Pelletier, K.R. (1977). *Mind as healer, mind as slayer.* New York: Delta.

Pelletier, K.R. (1978). *Toward a science of consciousness.* New York: Dell.

Pelletier, K.R. (1985). *A new age—problems and potential.* San Francisco: Robert Briggs.

Pfaff, D. (1968). Effects of temperature and time of day on time judgments. *Journal of Experimental Psychology, 76*, 419–422.

Piaget, J. (1970). *Structuralism.* New York: Harper Torchbook.

Plant, R. (1974). *Community and ideology*. London: Routledge & Kegan Paul.

Pollard, M.S. (1981). *Emotional expressiveness in cancer and noncancer patients*. Unpublished master's thesis, The Pennsylvania State University, University Park, PA.

Pratt, L. (1976). *Family structure and effective health behavior*. Boston: Houghton Mifflin.

Prigogine, I. (1976). Order through fluctuation: self-organization and social system. In E. Jantsch & C. H. Waddington (Eds.). *Evolution and consciousness*. Reading, MA: Addison-Wesley, pp. 93–133.

Prigogine, I. (1980). *From being to becoming*. San Francisco: W.H. Freeman.

Prigogine, I., Allen, P. M., & Herman, R. (1977). In E. Laszlo & J. Bierman (Eds.). *Goals in a global community: the original background papers for Goals for Mankind* (Vol. 1). New York: Pergamon Press, pp. 1–63.

Quinn, J. F. (1984). Therapeutic touch or energy exchange: testing the theory. *Advances in Nursing Science, 6* (2), 42–49.

Ravitz, L.J. (1962). History, measurement, and applicability of periodic changes in the electromagnetic field in health and disease. *Annals of the New York Academy of Science, 98,* 1144–1201.

Reiss D., & Oliveri, M.E. (1980). Family paradigm and family coping: a proposal for linking the family's intrinsic adaptive capacity to its response to stress. *Family Relations, 29,* 431–444.

Rodgers, J.A. (1972). Relationship between sociablility and personal space preference at two different times of day. *Perceptual and Motor Skills, 35,* 519–526.

Rogers, M.E. (1970). *An introduction to the theoretical basis of nursing*. Philadelphia: F.A. Davis.

Roy, C. (1984). Framework for classification systems development: progress and issues. In M.J. Kim, G.K. McFarland, & A.M. McLane, (Eds.). *Classification of nursing diagnoses*. St. Louis: The C.V. Mosby Co., pp. 26–40.

Roy, C., Rogers, M.E., Fitzpatrick, J.J., Newman, M.A., Orem, D., Feild, L., Stafford, M.J., Weber, S., Rossi, L., & Krekeler, K. (1982). Nursing diagnosis and nursing theory. In M.J. Kim & D.A. Moritz (Eds.). *Classification of nursing diagnoses*. New York: McGraw-Hill, pp. 214–278.

Ruberman, W., Weinblatt, E., Goldberg, J.D., & Chaudhary, B.S. (1984). Psychosocial influences on mortality after myocardial infarction. *The New England Journal of Medicine, 311,* 552–559.

Schmale, A., & Iker, H. (1966). The psychological setting of uterine cancer. *Annals of the New York Academy of Science, 125,* 807–813.

Seagel, S. (1982). Auditory perspective enlarges realm of hearing. *Brain-Mind Bulletin, 8*(1), 1–2.

Selye, H. (1956). *The stress of life*. New York: McGraw-Hill.

Sheldrake, R. (1981). *A new science of life: the hypothesis of formative causation*. Los Angeles: J.P. Tarcher.

Sheldrake, R. (1983). Testing a new science of life. *Investigations*, 1(1), 1–8.

Siffre, M. (1964). *Beyond time*. (H. Briffault, Trans.). New York: McGraw-Hill.

Smith, A. (1975). *Powers of mind*. New York: Random House.

Spinetta, J.J., Rigler, D., & Karon, M. (1974). Personal space as a measure of a dying child's senses of isolation. *Journal of Consulting and Clinical Psychology*, 42, 751–756.

Stanton, M.O. (1984). Fusion, compression, diversion and the working paradox: a theory of therapeutic/systematic change. *Family Process*, 23(2), 135–167.

Stephens, G.J. (1965). The time factor—should it control the patient's care? *American Journal of Nursing*, 65, 77–82.

Stone, H. (1978). *Holism: a new vision of man, a new vision of health*. Paper presented at conference on Holistic Perspectives: A Renaissance in Medicine and Health Care, Philadelphia, November 11–12.

Stone, H. (1985). *Embracing heaven and earth*. Mill Valley, CA: Delphi.

Stulman, J. (1972). The methodology of pattern. *Fields Within Fields*, 5(1), 7–41.

Teilhard de Chardin, P. (1959). *The phenomenon of man*. New York: Harper & Brothers.

Thomas, L. (1979). *The medusa and the snail*. New York: Viking Press.

Tiller, W.A. (1973). Some energy field observations of man and nature. In S. Krippner (Ed.). *Galaxies of life*. New York: Interface, pp. 71–111.

Tompkins, E.S. (1980). Effect of restricted mobility and dominance on perceived duration. *Nursing Research*, 29, 333–338.

Ubell, E. (1985). A world without disease. *Parade Magazine*, January 27.

Vaill, P.B. (1984–1985). Process wisdom for a new age. *Re-Vision*, 7(2), 39–49.

Vaughan, F.E. (1979). Transpersonal dimensions of psychotherapy. *Re-Vision*, 2(1), 26–29.

Von Bertalanffy, L. (1968). *General systems theory*. New York: Braziller.

Watson, L. (1976). *Gifts of unknown things*. New York: Simon & Schuster.

Watson, L. (1978). *Evolution and the unconscious*. Paper presented at symposium on New Dimensions of Consciousness, sponsored by Sufi Order in the West, New York, November 17–20.

Watson, L. (1979). *Lifetide: the biology of the unconscious*. New York: Simon & Schuster.

Weber, R. (1984). Compassion, rootedness, and detachment: their role in healing. A conversation with Dora Kunz. *Re-Vision*, 7(1), 76–82.

Welwood, J. (1978). The holographic paradigm and the structure of experience. *Re-Vision, 1*(3/4), 92–96.

West, M.C. (1984a). Community health assessment: the man-environment
interaction. *Journal of Community Health Nursing,* 1 (2), 89–97.

West, M. C. (1984b). *Patterns of health in mothers of developmentally disabled
children.* Unpublished master's thesis. The Pennsylvania University, University Park, PA.

Whyte, L.L. (1974). *The universe of experience.* New York: Harper & Row.

Wilbur, K. (1979). Spectrum psychology, Part *IV*: Into the transpersonal. *Re-
Vision, 2*(1), 65–72.

Wilbur, K. (1980). The pre/trans fallacy. *Re-Vision, 3* (2), 51–72.

Wilbur, K. (1983). *Up from Eden.* Boulder: Shambhala.

Young, A.M. (1976a). *The geometry of meaning.* San Francisco: Robert Briggs.

Young, A.M. (1976b). *The reflexive universe: evolution of consciousness.* San Francisco: Robert Briggs.

Index

A

Abse, D.W., 25
Absolute consciousness, 36
Ainsworth-Land, G., and Ainsworth-Land, V., 21, 84, 85, 89, 95
Allport, G., 91, 92
Ardell, D.B., 8
Awareness, higher levels of, 113–114

B

Bathrop, R.W., 25
Behnke, E.A., 59
Benner, P., 129
Bentov, Itzhak, 5, 22, 33, 34, 36, 37, 38, 63, 64, 65, 104
Biorhythms, 49–55
Blake, M.J.F., 50
Bohm, David, 5, 9, 11, 12, 13, 14, 15, 19, 29, 36, 58, 62–63, 71, 93, 109, 112, 130
Brandon, N., 113, 114
Brodie, John, 64
Byers, Paul, 60

C

Cancer, personality pattern of patient with, 25
Capra, F., 19, 87, 129
Cassandra: Radical Feminist Nurses Network, 98
Causality, 63
Causation, formative, Sheldrake's hypothesis of, 40
Change in nursing, cycles of, 84–86
Chetanananda, Swami, 102
Choosing in assessment, 74
Circadian cycles, 49–55
Client systems, 108, 109
Clients, relationships of health professionals with, expanding, 134
Cobey, V.E., 59, 61, 122
Colquhoun, W.P., 50
Communicating in assessment, 74
Community(ies)
application of new paradigm of health to, 107–134

Community(ies)—*continued*
energy fields in, 130–131
family, and individual as centers of consciousness, 32
movement in, 131
patterning of, 129–134
Community and family patterns of health and disease, 29–32
Community health, 131, 132
Condon, W.S., 55, 94
Conflict
nursing profession as center of, 80–81
and transformation, 103
Consciousness, 33–37
absolute, 36
Bentov's theory of evolution of, 5
centers of, individual, family, and community as, 32
evolution of, 34, 35, 37–41
pattern recognition as turning point in, 41–43
expanding
of family, 118–119
health as, formulation of concept of, 3–6
pattern of, 33–47
of self, 112–118
health as evolution of, 43–47
higher levels of, critical choices leading to, 47
highest level of, 65–67
integration of, via movement, 58–62
kinesthetic, 58–59
love and, 65–67
love as level of, 6
matter as manifestation of, 37
quantity and quality of, 35
time-space-movement as manifestation of, 48–67
transpersonal, 104
unfolding, 105
Cooperative inquiry, paradigm of, 94–95
Crisis causing change in pattern, 30–31
Critical choices leading to higher levels of consciousness, 47
Cycles of change in nursing, 84–86